THE Staying Healthy
—— Shopper's Guide ——

Feed Your Family Safely

by
Elson M. Haas, M.D.

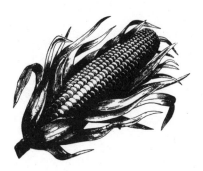

CELESTIALARTS
Berkeley, California

CELESTIALARTS

CELESTIAL ARTS PUBLISHING
P.O. Box 7123
Berkeley, California 94707

Celestial Arts titles are distributed in Canada by Ten Speed Canada, in the United Kingdom and Europe by Airlift Books, in South Africa by Real Books, in Australia by Simon & Schuster Australia, in New Zealand by Tandem Press, and in Southeast Asia by Berkeley Books.

Front cover photo by Tif Hunter© / Tony Stone Images
Back cover photo by Michael Buchanan
Cover design by Toni Tajima
Interior composition by Greene Design
Public domain illustrations courtesy of Dover Publications

Printed in the United States

Library Of Congress Card Catalog:
99-72207

1 2 3 4 5 6 7 8 / 05 04 03 02 01 00 99

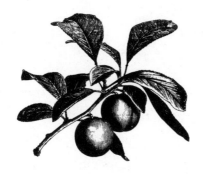

TABLE OF CONTENTS

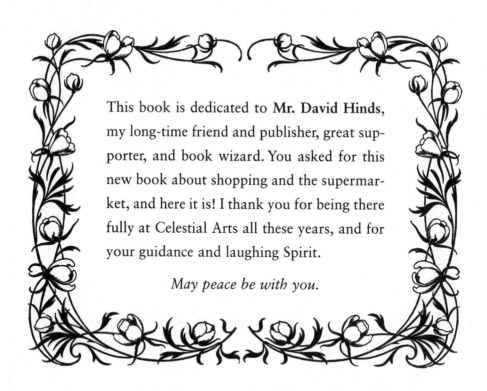

This book is dedicated to **Mr. David Hinds**, my long-time friend and publisher, great supporter, and book wizard. You asked for this new book about shopping and the supermarket, and here it is! I thank you for being there fully at Celestial Arts all these years, and for your guidance and laughing Spirit.

May peace be with you.

Acknowledgements to My Capable Co-workers:

Nancy Faass—For your expert contribution through research, writing support, design ideas, and going that extra mile when it really counts. You are a shining jewel and wonderful to work with! Thank you.

Bethany S. ArgIsle, CEO ArgIsle Enterprises <www.ARGISLE.com> To the "Queen of User-Friendly" and inter-networker, thank you for your creative book development, inspired editing, design guidance, and your continued support in making the Staying Healthy books over 20 years. You are one in a billion!

Also, I would like to commend:

Mark Squire of Good Earth Natural Foods since 1975, specializing in organic products (Fairfax, CA <www.ge@ap.net>) and long-time CCOF member—for your review and insights on the Chapter 7.

To **Gene Shaparenko** of Aqua Technology (San Jose, CA) and **Michael Davis** of The Water Store (Greenbrae, CA) for your informed reviews on Chapter 8.

To **PANNA** (Pesticide Action Network of North America) and **EWG** (Earth Working Group) for your knowledgable support and great information. Their staff and web sites, <www.panna.org> and <www.ewg.org> were very helpful.

To **Norman Rolfe** for your industriousness and helpful research.

How to Use This Book

When you go shopping for your weekly groceries, you're faced with an overwhelming number of little choices that all add up to your health. *The Staying Healthy Shopper's Guide* was written to help you make those choices based on solid information.

In Chapters 1 through 4, we take a closer look at the causes for concern about our food supply—the everyday toxic risks of our most common foods, including many of the items you'll find in any grocery store. I provide scientific and government support for these concerns, including data you rarely see in the mainstream media.

This information tends to be more environmentally explicit and intense than any of my previous books. So, if you want to explore the basic facts regarding the widespread pollution of the Earth and our food supply, you will want to read the book from cover to cover. I believe it will motivate you to make positive changes in your food choices and lifestyle habits.

Chapters 5 through 12 offer solutions. If you are already aware of the toxicity of our foods, or if you have a weak stomach or psyche for negative data, I encourage you to turn directly to these later chapters for lighter, more positive information. Simply begin at Chapter 5 and read from that point. Check out the many charts that are included to assist you in planning your forays into the garden, the market, and the refrigerator. You will also find helpful resources at the end of many chapters.

The evidence continues to suggest that pesticides, additives, and environmental toxins pose a threat to our health, so for my own family, I buy organically-grown foods and products, filtered water, and nutritional supplements. It is my hope to inspire you to make wise choices to stay healthy and feed your family safely.

Be well.

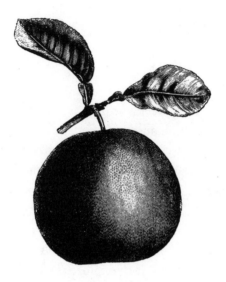

*An organic apple a day
keeps the doctor away.*

CHAPTER ONE

What We Need to Know Before We Shop

Most of us puzzle over the labels on products in the grocery store—What should we buy? What's really healthy? What's safe? These are important questions because what we eat is one of the major influences on how healthy we are now and how healthy we'll be in the future.

What we eat not only affects how we feel today, but also how we will feel 10 to 20 years from now. Generally, our health evolves (or declines) gradually over time. Physical problems actually grow out of our daily habits and exposures: what we eat; whether we get enough exercise and rest; the degree to which we manage stress; and the load of toxins and microbes on our body systems. Conditions such as cancer and cardiovascular disease, for example, frequently develop over two or three decades.

Most of us are reluctant to change our bad habits, because we seem to get away with them. We may be eating poorly—eating junk food, skipping meals, overeating, eating on the run, or eating at the wrong times for optimum use of fuel and our own bio-clock—but we don't really connect it with how we feel. If we are not tuned into our energy level, we won't notice much difference from hour to hour or from day to day. Thus, we may not equate what we eat now with how we may feel later in the day. Nor will we have a way to compare how we feel today with how we *could* feel.

Speaking Personally

Did you ever wonder how you would feel if you took a break for a week, ate really healthfully, and took a vacation from the foods that drain your energy? Speaking personally, until I did my first ten-day juice fast back in 1975, I couldn't make any kind of comparison. Sure, I had days when I felt pretty good, but the rest of the time, I just walked around in my sluggish, semiproductive state—and I didn't even realize how low my energy was until I began experiencing a more energized and vital way of being.

After my first juice fast, I realized that I needed to break some lifelong habits and make some permanent changes in order to truly fulfill my potential. I thought about (or projected) what I might look and feel like at age sixty if I kept eating and living the way I was. I sensed that I could affect my future by what I did in the present, and that insight changed my life. As a friend of mine used to say, "Don't correct your past, correct your future." And my focus on Preventive Medicine began with this awareness.

In all honesty, it's an ongoing process for me, as food and its preparation is one of my passions, hobbies, and an addictive habit. Also, I travel frequently, which has many challenges, and I have two school-age children, so there is always plenty of food and snacks around the house for them, as well as parties and other food-centered activities. So, I periodically fast or do a cleansing diet to keep my body lighter and in balance. I am committed to this at least twice yearly. (Read about this in my first book, *Staying Healthy with the Seasons*).

Our energy, our health, and our physical body are the result of our habits and lifestyle, as well as our genetic makeup and our early conditioning and exposures. Shifting any lifestyle habit will create a different result. The idea of actually becoming renewed—trimmer, more vital, healthier. Shifting our habits can make it happen!

We rarely rethink our day-to-day habits, because we don't realize that each little action can influence our overall health. Change can be difficult, because for most of us, lifelong habits, such as eating processed foods, are so pervasive that we don't even question them. Most of us change only in response to a crisis, which is why a crisis can often be a blessing in disguise. However, if we wait until we are seriously ill, when physical damage has occurred, then not only won't we be able to reach our higher potential, our health crisis may be irreversible and quite expensive.

Let me share my own experience of some habits I was able to change, which I believe helped me not only to be happier and healthier immediately, but also influenced my health over my lifetime. When I was growing up, it seemed as though I lived on peanut butter and jelly smeared on fluffy white bread, milk, and potato chips—a meal high in fat, high in sugar, and high in calories. Later, I graduated to the local deli for cheeseburgers, fries, and colas for lunch—fat, more fat, and sugar. Throughout my childhood, breakfasts were sugar-coated cereals with milk and more sugar. Dinners were meat and potatoes, bread and butter, sometimes salad, and always dessert, plus a big glass of fat-laden whole cow's milk. And before bed, I routinely had more milk and cookies or ice cream milkshakes. I was overweight, congested, and allergic, and had at least three to four colds a year.

As a teenager, I worked in my family's Blue Dot Market in Detroit. I enjoyed anything I wanted from any department in the store—especially from our eight-foot-long candy counter. My entire family was overweight, even though we all worked hard and I played sports almost every day.

When I went away to school, I dined in college cafeterias and fraternity houses and chose mostly eggs, bacon, and fried bread for breakfast, a hearty lunch, and a huge dinner. Later, during medical school, I ate in hospital cafeterias—donuts, burgers, and potatoes were among my favorites. It wasn't until I became a doctor that I realized that my food choices were the cause of my weight problems and my sluggish energy. It *did* matter what I put into my body, because it became part of me. So, I ate more fruits and vegetables and less of the junk I was used to. To my surprise, these changes left me feeling nourished and satisfied and—presto, chango—I began to look and feel tremendously better, trimmer, and healthier. As I shifted more of my habits and made different choices, I not only lost weight, but I became less congested and less allergic, and continued to feel great. I have maintained these improved habits over the years, and I enjoy good health today.

NUTRITION

Nutrition is an important key to preventing disease. And that is the essence of *The Staying Healthy Shopper's Guide*. My goal is to provide you with the information upon which to base your daily decisions about what you eat and where you shop. This book offers a practical, healthful guide to help you shop, cook, and eat in ways that can make a measurable difference in your life.

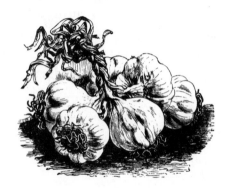

Most of us are dependent on our local supermarket because we have little access to farm-fresh produce or organic meats. So we need to become highly informed shoppers by learning some important basics.

Keys to Proactive Shopping

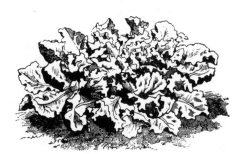

- How and when to select and prepare the freshest produce

- When to buy organic

- Which products to get in the health food section

- The hidden *unlabeled* ingredients in everyday foods

- How to read food labels

- The safest approach to food additives

- Foods best avoided to maintain health

Following these shopping guidelines will enhance your health and also help you avert the medical problems that occur from chronic exposure to pesticides and chemicals that are being used on our food and farmlands today. The ideas in this book actually reflect an important aspect of Preventive Medicine: that good nutrition is more effective in *preventing* disease than in treating problems *after* they occur. Your potential for good health will be optimized if you consume a nutritious diet and also exercise regularly, get enough sleep, manage stress, and keep a positive attitude toward life—these are the five key areas of Preventive Medicine.

The Temptation of Processed Food

In contrast to the goal of a clean, simple diet is the temptation of rich food. The magic of technology entices us with an endless array of snazzy products—sweet and easy, effortless and perhaps addictive—and distracts us from the whole, fresh fuel our body truly needs.

The supermarket, and now the huge natural food stores, are the culmination of modern technology and the industrial food revolution. They are the super storefronts, showcasing all the "miracle" products—just waiting for your reaction to their newest TV commercial or magazine ad. When we walk down the aisles of the average mega-supermarket, we are tempted by colorful bags, boxes, and jars full of exotic products, strange and familiar produce from all around the globe, a myriad of instant convenience foods, and a variety of intriguing new products. Not only are many of these products unnecessary for our health, their manufacture is often unhealthy for our planetary environment. In a free enterprise system, government can't really control how many of these unnecessary and toxic products are being produced and which additives are introduced into our food. There is no limit on food manufacturing—corporations large and small can create wonder colas, super sugary snacks, and refined, devitalized foods without substance, while agribusiness can market produce laced with pesticides that are clearly not all healthy for us.

We can choose with our spending dollars; one dollar is our vote.

The message is "Buyer beware." But the health guidelines we are taught in school, in the news, and by our doctors stand in contrast with what is actually available to us when we go out to shop. Of course, we shouldn't be influenced by fancy advertising, clever packaging, and enhanced flavors. And although we can't control the tempting nature of these rich foods, we can control ourselves, or can we? If we want to reap the benefits of a healthy diet, we must learn to turn away from the seduction of empty calories or foods laden with fat and chemicals.

Back to the Earth in the 21st Century

Have you focused on a reconnection with the Earth and a more natural approach to health? This is a trend I promote and support in my preventive medical practice, my writing, and my own lifestyle. Many of us are eating more naturally again, even growing some of our own food or shopping at farmers' markets, and using more wholesome, less chemicalized products from the natural foods stores. I personally have gone for years without needing very much from the supermarket—by eating mostly fresh fruits, vegetables, whole grains, sprouts, beans, nuts and seeds, and buying organically-grown produce and organically-made products. It is a little less convenient and a little more expensive, but I consider this extra time and money a worthy tradeoff for a healthy lifestyle and a potentially more vital future.

General Concerns

Important research shows that there are good reasons to be concerned about our food supply: the loss of nutrients that results from modern methods of farming; polluted water; depleted soil; the high level of chemicals in everyday consumer foodstuffs; the overprocessing of foods; exposure to harmful microbes; and the toxicity of animal products.

But why a whole book just to buy the "right" kind of peanut butter or a "better" bread for sandwiches? How much does it really matter?

This book was written to help clarify the issues at hand, to motivate you, and to provide you with information so that you can make your own best decisions. (Consider keeping track of your changes, however few or many, however small or grand; realize that your evolution may progress and then backtrack, before you make long-term habit changes.)

Let's take a closer look at how our food is grown, how chemicals and pollutants enter the agricultural food chain from both industrial and farming practices, how and why food is processed, and what is added or removed before it gets to our table. Chemicals in our diets and our immediate environment are of major concern, especially in relationship to chronic, serious diseases such as cancer and leukemia. Staying healthy involves minimizing the toxins in our food and in our environment.

Eating a clean, whole-foods diet that contains a minimum of pesticides and additives will decrease the toxic load on the body and enhance our physical vitality.

At this point, you may be wondering if our foods really are so chemically laden, why don't we know about it? Surely our government protects, or at least, informs us. Yes and no. We may be consuming literally thousands of chemicals in our food that result from farming and food processing. The Food and Drug Administration defines many of these chemicals as "indirect additives," for which no labeling is required. But the quantity is overwhelming. In 1995, the USDA reported that more than two billion pounds of pesticides were used in U.S. agriculture. When the FDA tested produce at random, they found pesticide residues on *two-thirds* of the food tested. And although these chemicals are legal, many of them are still untested for human consumption.

Luckily, a healthy body can handle much of this. However, the cumulative burden of chemical exposure is a crucial issue for most of us, whether we know it or not. Our health could be at risk due to the persistent bombardment of chemical stressors, some of which we knowingly ingest and many others of which we are not yet aware.

I am also very concerned about the chemicals used in raising livestock for food and the sprays with which growers fumigate their harvested foods (which accounts for 20% of pesticide use.) And although fish can be a healthy diet choice, water pollution increases our chemical intake if we consume seafood regularly. (There are also other sources of exposure in which the toxins tend to be more concentrated, such as the chemical treatment of cotton clothing and furniture, the outgassing of synthetic carpeting or paints, or the chemicals in cigarette smoke exposure. I will save these concerns for another book.)

Chemical contaminants slip into our food chain—perhaps because few of us really take them seriously. For example, there are more than 3,000 "direct additives" legally allowed in our food, identified on the labels. We tend to think that chemical exposure is no big deal, and the industry suggests that "everything goes better with chemistry." However, I believe we need to send a different message:

Use as few chemicals as possible and preferably no toxic chemicals at all.

Periodically, we also have to cope with food contaminated by germs—pathogenic bacteria, viruses, parasites, or molds. We know historically, and most of us know by experience, that unfriendly microbes in our body can make us very ill (and occasionally can be devastating). In mass food production, antibiotics are used to suppress microbes; this adds another class of chemicals to our food intake. If our goal is food free from chemicals, greater care must be taken to avoid the contamination of our food with microorganisms. The E. coli infections due to unpasteurized apple juice and meat-packing practices resulting in tainted hamburgers are examples we don't want repeated.

As part of our technological society, the agricultural industry is always trying to improve on Nature. Food products are supposed to get better, bigger, and grow faster. But Nature requires our interaction and patience. We need to be cautious in our selection of food because some of the current practices in the food industry are still essentially unproven. This includes genetically-engineered products (produce, meat, and milk), the use of hormones (in meat and milk production), and food irradiation. Generally, labeling is not yet required for most of these practices. There needs to be more research, so that we can use these products with the assurance of safety. **Until we have more information on their long-term safety, I recommend caution in their use.**

The Staying Healthy Shopper's Guide provides an overview of why processed foods and food additives are used, the most important additives to avoid, and those that don't appear to pose a risk. I will also look at the loss of nutritive value through food processing. Organic foods and whole fresh foods typically have higher levels of nutrients, and therefore are most ideal for us to consume as the main component of our diet.

Choosing Optimum Nutrition

The real message of this book is to use fewer processed foods and return to a more natural diet. I encourage you not to depend on convenience foods. Work toward consuming at least 70% of your diet from fresh and whole-food choices such as fruits, vegetables, whole grains, beans, sprouts, nuts and seeds, low-fat dairy products, and some animal proteins, if desired. With every step you take to prepare food, there will inevitably be some loss of vitality and nutrients. There are so many wholesome meals and snacks that can be eaten fresh or easily prepared. Try to be sure your food is clean, consciously raised, and organic as possible. How do you live now? How do you want to live in the future?

Everything we eat affects our health and vitality; every agricultural practice comes back to us in the animals and produce we consume. And every day we have the opportunity to make healthier choices, consume fewer chemicals, and eat more vital food. We have to decide, however, that it's worth the time, energy, and money.

I hope this book will encourage you to follow a healthy lifestyle and eat more wholesome, seasonal, and natural foods, free of chemical additives and contaminants which will result in greater energy and vitality, more enthusiasm for life, quality aging, and all the other benefits of staying healthy.

Be well by living well.

—Dr. Elson

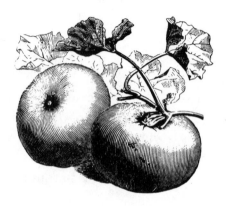

CHAPTER TWO

Why Should We Care About Chemicals in Our Food?

◆

The health of the Earth and the health of our bodies are aligned. When the Earth is compromised, none of us can be entirely healthy. Pollution is now so prevalent on our planet that it affects us all, no matter where we live. Industrial chemicals have surrounded and invaded our entire world. Of course, some of these chemicals also have a beneficial role in our consumer-oriented society.

The agricultural industry has worked diligently to find new ways to increase crop yields and develop new products. Many of these developments could not have occurred without creative new discoveries in the field of chemistry. But there has been a price—our health, and thus, our future. We all need to be aware of the impact of agricultural and industrial chemicals in our food and water. They affect our personal health and the health of our children and they impact our local and global environments.

Common Chemical Exposures

In this chapter, I discuss some of the many ways that chemicals get into our food and water supply. Exposures come from a variety of sources:

- Pesticides and fertilizers

- Industrial pollutants, such as chemicals and heavy metals

- Food additives

- Contaminants associated with the processing of foods

- Chemicals and drugs used in raising livestock

Pesticides and fertilizers: Chapter Three will focus on pesticides and agricultural pollution. Simply, this is likely the riskiest technological toxin exposure we have,

REASONS TO BE A PROACTIVE SHOPPER: CHEMICALS AND TOXINS IN OUR FOOD

How Many of These Are on Your Shopping List?

DIRECT ADDITIVES TO FOODS
- **Labeled additives** such as sugars, salt, sulfites, preservatives, etc.
- **Additives listed by general category,** not required to be identified by name, include artificial food colors and artificial food flavorings

POLLUTANTS: Unintentional (typically not labeled)
- **Pollutants, chemicals, and pesticide residues** from the air, water, or soil
- **Toxic industrial wastes** in fertilizer that contaminate ground and surface water and soil (270 million pounds from 1990 to 1995—all unlisted, not on fertilizer labels)
- **Toxic concentrations of minerals** in the soil or water (selenium, sodium chloride, and nitrates)
- **Toxic heavy metals** in the water that accumulate in soil, water, and in the tissue of fish and shellfish (lead, mercury, arsenic, cadmium, chromium)

UNLISTED CHEMICALS used in farming and processing (but not on the label)
- **Pesticides** sprayed on soil, plants, trees, and crops
- **Equipment cleaners** such as bleaches, detergents, rinses, etc.
- **Food sprays** such as mold inhibitors on fruits, pesticides and gases applied before shipping
- **Chemicals** contained in other ingredients, used in the preparation of processed foods, such as MSG, toxins in lard, pesticide residues in food waxes
- **Chemicals given to animals** include antibiotics, insecticide sprays, pesticides in feed, steroids and hormones to stimulate growth, sedatives and other drugs used for slaughter.

MICROBES
In the fields and orchards
In shipping from the farm or factory
In mass processing and preparation
In the slaughter and packing houses
In shipping from the factory to families
From improper storage in the store or at home

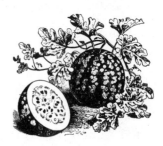

Kitchen counters and sponges, refrigerator bins
In restaurant preparation or from food handlers
In the grocery store, at deli counters and salad bars,
  in free sampling and open-air displays

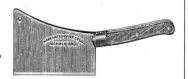

FOOD PROCESSES RESULTING IN LOSS OF NUTRITIVE VALUE

- **Milling of grains** such as wheat, rice, oats, and barley to create "instant" foods, which removes essential nutrients such as the bran (an important source of fiber) and the seed (a source of essential vitamins, minerals, and oils)
- **Refining,** for example, when sugar cane is processed to make white sugar, the nutritious portion is discarded
- **Overprocessing of food** is the prolonged and high-temperature heating of foods, chemical cleaning, and automated meat processing
- **Synthesizing** is a process by which artificial foods are created, such as olestra and sweeteners. These are low in nutrients and potentially toxic.
- **Artificial processes,** for example, making honey by feeding bees sugar water does not create the same nutrient-rich honey as that derived from free-roaming bees that collect flower pollen and nectar
- **Storage methods,** such as canning, freezing, and packaging, can decrease the vitamin content of foods

ADDITIONAL UNLISTED FOOD PROCESSES AND ADDITIVES

- **Genetically-engineered foods** (which do not yet require labeling). Engineered foods include vegetables with built-in pesticides; coffee beans with altered caffeine content; and produce manipulated to extend shelflife, such as corn, wheat, peppers, and fruits
- **Genetically-engineered hormones** such as the engineered growth hormones (like BGH) that increase the milk production of dairy cows (no labeling requirement exists)
- **Unlisted additives from processing** meat products can contain bone, bone marrow, and even spinal cord and lower nutrient levels; earlier methods also included bone
- **Food irradiation** is frequently unlisted and may be more commonplace than we know; its risks to our health are still an unknown. It is used on produce, spices, and animal meats.

and the most insidious. Nearly all of us are exposed daily unless we take rigorous precautions.

Pesticides play a complex role in agribusiness. Pesticides make it possible for enormous amounts of food to be raised efficiently, yet they place a major toxic burden on the Earth and its human and animal populations. In 1995, more than 5 billion pounds of pesticides were sold worldwide ($35 billion worth!), with more than 1 billion pounds in the U.S. (valued at $10 billion!). In addition to conventional pesticides, 250 million pounds of other toxic chemicals were used as pesticides and herbicides, such as petroleum products and sulfur. These pesticides remain on our food, and FDA inspections have found *legal* residues on two-thirds of the food sampled, while imported produce typically has even higher levels.

The kinds of damage that can result from pesticides have been well documented in workplace exposure and in animal studies. *The Handbook of Pesticide Toxicology* requires four volumes to describe all the harmful effects, in more than 1,200 pages (Hayes and Law, 1991). And the occupational handbook, *Human Health Effects of Pesticides* (M. C. Keifer, Ed., 1997), is more than 400 pages and cites hundreds of research studies. Although these exposures are stronger than those we receive through our food and water each day, it is important to note that cancer, leukemia, and other degenerative diseases are often linked to much lower-level exposures.

Industrial pollutants: Whether we live in large cities, sprawling suburbs, or rural communities, industrial pollutants typically enter our drinking water through ground waters and our food supply. These include chemical waste products such as solvents and gasoline, dioxins and PCBs, asbestos and plastics. Toxic metals that include lead, mercury, arsenic, aluminum, cadmium, and chromium, also contaminate our waters. Recent testing suggests that mercury, for example, may now contaminate all ocean tuna. Radioactive waste also contaminates the oceans in all parts of the globe and affects most sea life on the planet.

In the U.S. alone, the Great Lakes and more than 16,000 waterways are polluted, as well as almost 8,000 miles of shoreline. Finding a clean source of seafood becomes a major problem when you consider that most sealife being tested show traces of mercury, DDT, and other industrial chemicals. Almost 9 million tons of oil is estimated to enter the ocean each year, as well as an estimated 14 billion pounds of garbage. Between 1990 and 1994, chemical plants, pulp mills, steel factories, and other manufacturing industries dumped more than 1 billion pounds of toxic chemicals into American rivers, lakes, streams, bays, and coastal waters. During this same period, an estimated 450 million pounds of chemical waste was flushed by factories and through sewage treatment plants into our waters (Environmental Working Group).

Food additives: Over 12,000 chemicals are used in the production of our food. Some are used intentionally during the various stages of growing, harvesting, preparing, processing, packing, and shipping. Many are present as intentional or "direct" additives and others as accidental or "indirect" contaminants. As of 1995, there was toxicity information available on 54% of the food additives in use, and complete health-risk assessments were available for only 5% of food additives. Billions of pounds of additives are used in processed meats alone in the United States.

The food industry uses about 3,000 different food additives in a wide variety of packaged and preserved foods. These range from added vitamins and minerals to emulsifiers, buffers, natural and artificial flavorings and colorings, and large amounts of salt and sugar. The average American consumes over 150 pounds of food additives a year, including about 130 pounds of sweeteners, totaling almost 40 billion pounds in 1995. In addition, we each typically consume about 10 to 15 pounds of salt, plus another 5 to 10 pounds of added flavorings, preservatives, and colored dyes.

Contaminants (indirect): The cleaning products used during the manufacturing process may show up in the final product we consume. This is usually in small amounts and not as big a risk as other areas of food processing.

Chemicals can enter our food during any stage: from the soil while growing, after harvesting, during processing, and before packing, shipping, or storage. Soil contaminants such as nitrates or selenium may be absorbed, in addition to the sometimes toxic additives found in commercial fertilizers. Changes in the nature of a plant or animal product due to genetic engineering or from hormones are not yet required to be listed on the label.

During shipping and storage, a variety of chemical cleaners, food sprays, and fumigants are used. Unlisted additives can also enter our food supply during processing, including petroleum waxes on fruits and vegetables, sulfur and other preservatives on dried fruits (some listed and some not), and additives such as MSG contained in the ingredients of precooked products. Meats may contain organic contaminants, such as bits of bone from processing and other less pleasant residues.

Chemicals and drugs used in raising animals: This should be one of our greatest concerns—the amount of chemicals used in raising poultry and livestock while they are housed in cramped quarters under inhumane conditions. Chemicals in feed, growth enhancers, and antibiotics may contaminate the meat byproducts. Yet none of the chemicals or drugs used is required to appear on the label. The antibiotic levels used in animals for market involves 20 tons each year (given orally, as implants, and as injections). Antibacterials, topical antimicrobials, and insecticides are used in the feed, the living quarters, and directly on the animals themselves. Hormones are given to speed their growth and increase milk production. Steroids or steroid-like hormones are given to increase muscle mass. Additives and pesticides can be found in the feed. During the slaughtering process, sedatives such as beta-blockers, or other drugs are administered. *It is not surprising that researchers fear this source of contamination may ultimately be among the worst in our food supply.*

Cause for Concern?

It is the job of the U.S. Food and Drug Administration (FDA) to carry out the laws written for consumer protection. One of the legal mandates of the FDA is the Delaney Clause, which prohibits the human use of chemicals found, through research, to cause cancer in animals. Clearly, if a chemical or drug causes illness in rats or mice, it may also be dangerous to humans. But we have almost no information about the effects on humans of most chemicals, such as food additives, and in particular, the effects that occur over a lifetime of exposure. We do know there is a higher incidence of cancer among farmers and farm workers who use pesticides, but their exposure is probably much higher than that of the average food consumer. Those who profit from technochemical development would like us to believe that the constant exposure to tiny amounts of these toxic materials poses little or no risk.

In this chapter, you will learn how chemicals pervade what you eat, and what kinds of health concerns this raises. Later in the book, I will discuss how to reduce your intake of chemicalized foods and how to minimize the long-term effects from having ingested chemicals throughout your life. I'll also offer practical suggestions for a realistic, healthful way to feed yourself and your family.

As the Earth becomes more and more polluted, so do our bodies. Today, many of our most common diseases are environmental in nature, involving our interaction with our surroundings. Some of this chemical exposure is avoidable, but in many cases, we are at the mercy of others, of their conscience (and unconsciousness)—past, present, and future.

The degree to which we are likely to be harmed by the detrimental effects of food chemicals depends on a number of factors. These include our general state of health, how we handle stress, whether or not we use other drugs—alcohol, tobacco, caffeine, prescription and non—and whether or not we generally eat a high-fat diet or a lot of junk food. Are we in generally good health? When we think about our vulnerability to the harmful consequences of chemicals, it is useful to compare it with our vulnerability to germs; some microorganisms are strong enough to cause problems even in the healthiest person, but most germs generally need a weakened host or compromised immune system in order to take hold and multiply in the body. The same principle holds true for the hazards of food chemicals.

Very few of the studies on either pesticides or food additives have looked at multiple exposures or chemical interactions, despite the fact that many crops and many processed foods may contain half-a-dozen or more questionable chemicals, all in a single product.

One example of these chemical interactions is the formation of trihalomethanes (THMs), many of which are carcinogenic. THMs are formed when chlorine or fluoride combines with a hydrocarbon, such as gasoline or other petroleum products, creating toxic and carcinogenic chlorinated hydrocarbons. Both chlorine and fluoride are added to most municipal water supplies, so the danger posed by THMs is very real. Another example is the nitrosamines. These are formed when nitrites or nitrates in foods or in water react with other organic acids in our body or in the foods we eat to form the highly carcinogenic nitrosamines. Nitrites are typically found in everyday foods such as hot dogs and other luncheon meats.

Can we assume in our free-market society that agribusiness is looking out for our health? Or is their responsibility to market their products for a stockholder's profit? (And when some chemicals are found to be too toxic for continued use, they are sold to Third World countries to use on their crops and then return to the U.S. as imports, which is about a third of our produce.)

SPECIFIC HEALTH ISSUES REGARDING CHEMICALS IN OUR FOOD

- **Lack of research data:** *The hidden danger is in repeated small exposures over time, about which we still have very little real data.*
- **Not enough information:** *Insufficient information exists about potentially toxic interactions of the many chemicals in the environment and in our bodies.*
- **Chemicals that interact and form new toxins:** *Chemicals do interact with each other. Various industrial chemicals may combine in nature, in products, or within our body as new chemicals, which can be even more toxic than the original.*
- **Our body's inability to cope:** *Because our ancestors did not live in a chemical environment, we do not have the enzymes necessary to break down or metabolize and eliminate these synthetic chemicals.*
- **Chemicals remain in our body:** *Chemicals can accumulate in our body tissues and become a source of ongoing toxicity. Chemicals stored in our body fat and other tissues may be released regularly and continually into our system over time, thus generating an ongoing toxic effect.*
- **Repeated exposures:** *When repeated insults occur from the same or similar chemicals, they can damage our cells and tissues, endangering our health. Multiple chemical exposures can lead to chronic disease, such as cancer. Harmful effects to the nervous system and to reproductive health may be a more common threat than we realize.*
- **Undisclosed exposure:** *The majority of the chemicals in our foods are not disclosed on the label, and thus making informed choices difficult.*
- **Testing falls short:** *Because testing looks primarily at very high exposures, we lack information on the toxic threshold level of many chemicals in humans—the level at which damage begins to occur.* **We don't really know how much is too much.**
- **Exposure and the individual:** *Dose and response are highly individual—based on many factors, such as age, size, and metabolism. Legally allowable exposure levels for both food additives and pesticides are based on the tolerance of a healthy adult male. Women, children, the elderly, and people who are already ill are not taken into consideration.*
- **Delayed effects:** *Researchers found that when infant animals were given neurotoxic doses of food additives they failed to show overt signs of distress. Damage to the nervous system and vision was not evident until the animal approached adulthood.*
- **Interplay of chemicals and immune function:** *The condition of our health and immunity is very important. When we are stressed or overly fatigued, we become more vulnerable to chemical insults.*

DAMAGE FROM CHEMICALS IN OUR FOOD

Agricultural chemicals and industrial pollutants both interact with and contaminate life. Some can even destroy life when they become concentrated enough. The greatest causes for concern are the chemicals that contaminate our soil and our water, and that are added to our food. Pesticides, fungicides, herbicides, and preservatives become part of our food during the various stages, from before growth to processing. There is an overwhelming body of research that links these toxins with serious conditions such as liver disease, cancer, damage to the nervous system, hormone imbalances, and even death. Specific pollutants may create additional health risks regionally, such as the water contamination in Louisiana, or the heavy chemical use in agricultural areas of California and Florida.

Chemicals with highly toxic potential are categorized by the EPA (Environmental Protection Agency) and researchers according to their harmful effects on the body. These include:

- Cancer-promoting toxins (carcinogens)—chemicals that increase the incidence of cancer

- Mutagenic toxins—chemicals that can alter genetic makeup

- Reproductive toxins—affects fertility in both men and women

- Developmental toxins—harmful to the unborn and to growing children

- Endocrine-disrupters—toxins that mimic hormones and can cause cancer

- Nerve toxins—causing adverse effects to the nervous system

Pesticides, pollutants, and agricultural chemicals have additional harmful effects:

- Immediate adverse effects from direct exposure

- Development of chemical sensitivity and other immune disorders

- Worsening of health in those with chronic conditions

- Problems of liver and kidney function

- Long-term or latent effects on the average person

- Negative impact on wildlife

- Damage to the environment

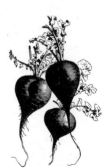

Cancer-promoting Toxins

The EPA labeling actually identifies some agricultural chemicals in current use as "probable human carcinogens." At least 107 different active ingredients in pesticides have been found to cause cancer in animals or humans; of these, 71 are still in use *on food crops* (National Campaign for Pesticide Policy Reform). Food additives documented to cause cancer in animal studies include artificial food coloring, BHA and BHT, nitrates, and saccharin.

There are two stages in the process by which chemicals can cause disease, particularly cancer. The first is through direct irritation to the cells and tissues of the body. A chemical that is a potential carcinogen (termed an *initiator*) may actually bind to the DNA within the cell, altering its structure and potential for normal duplication.

When our immune system is weakened, or when there are just too many chemical insults for our body to handle, a second stage of tissue breakdown can occur. Certain toxins (*cancer promoters*) may then stimulate the development of a growing malignancy.

Mutagenic Toxins

These are chemicals in our food that can alter genetic makeup and can have an adverse effect on human development when the exposure occurs during pregnancy. Many pesticides, known as endocrine disrupters, can affect not only the reproductive system, but genetic makeup as well. Depending on the types of hormones present during fetal development, specific genes can be permanently turned on or off, *just by changing the amount of the hormones involved.* Chemicals—some pesticides and fumigants—that mimic human hormones, such as estradiol and estrogen, can actually initiate the genetic activity that determines how cells will function for the entire life of an unborn person. Even extremely small amounts can lead to dramatic changes in the way genes function, a process known as *genetic imprinting*. When manmade chemicals that are consumed in food or water appear at the wrong times and in the wrong amounts, unpredictable outcomes can occur.

Reproductive Toxins

A number of adverse effects on the reproductive system have been linked to the influence of toxic chemicals, particularly pesticides. These effects were first noticed in birds: male birds became sterile, eggs developed with damaged shells, and birth defects occurred more frequently. And now frogs and other wildlife worldwide are experiencing an increase in birth malformations. Researchers have linked reproductive damage specifically to pesticides, heavy metal pollutants, and a number of chemicals, including dioxin.

Studies of human reproductive patterns have also shown compromised reproductive capacity due to chemical pollutants. Human sperm counts have been declining worldwide over much of this century. Danish researchers reported this decline in 1992, based on the analysis of 61 different studies. A 1997 report showed a sperm production decline in the United States over the past 50 years of about 1.5% a year. Experts blame persistent organic pollutants, ranging from pesticides such as DDT to industrial chemicals like PCBs.

In women, exposure to pesticides has been associated with problems of infertility, spontaneous abortion, miscarriage, stillbirth, premature births, and birth defects (*Designer Poisons*, Moses, 1995). Studies conducted in China and in the U.S. found that women working in agriculture and exposed to pesticides during pregnancy had children with higher rates of leukemia. At least four other studies have linked pesticide exposure during pregnancy with the increased incidence of brain cancer in children. Also, an increased frequency of miscarriages occurs in women who drink municipal waters with higher amounts of chlorine-based THMs.

Certain food additives have also been associated with reproductive problems. For example caffeine, found in colas, chocolate, coffee, and tea, may interfere with reproduction and affect developing fetuses. Experiments on lab animals linked caffeine to birth defects such as cleft palates, missing fingers and toes, and skull malformations.

Is it possible that we have overlooked the extent to which we are altering everything around us, and the ways in which those alterations are coming back to us?

Developmental Toxins

Developmental toxins can cause a number of different toxic effects on both unborn and young children. For example, endocrine-disrupting chemicals such as pesticides can affect the hormone levels in a developing fetus. This suggests how potent and potentially dangerous these chemicals can be. The potential effects of chemicals are also a concern with growing children. Their ability to fight infections and detoxify chemicals is less well developed than adults. Generally, young children tend to eat more fruits and vegetables than adults, thus taking in a greater toxic burden in proportion to their body weight.

The Food Quality Protection Act requires the EPA to reconsider data on the sensitivity of children and others with special needs. In the past, pesticide tolerances have been based on the metabolism of a typical healthy adult male weighing 155 pounds. The National Academy of Sciences has pointed out that standard risk assessments may seriously underestimate potential harm, particularly for infants and children.

Research shows that the occurrence of brain tumors in children has escalated by 30% in the past fifteen years, and childhood malignancies and leukemia are up by more than 10%. At least nine studies have noted an increase in cancers among children whose parents were exposed to pesticides in the workplace. Nineteen other studies found links between pesticide use and childhood cancers. Children living in homes where home and garden pesticides were used were at least twice as likely to develop cancer. In some of the studies, home use of pesticides increased risk as much as seven times (NCAMP). In addition, adverse effects on the nervous system can occur from even low-level exposure to pesticides or chemicals in foods.

Endocrine Disrupters

Certain pesticides have been found to lengthen the estrogen cycle, prolonging the body's exposure to estrogen and significantly increasing the possibility of cancer. DDT is the most well-known of this class of pesticides that have been linked to increased cancer incidence. Although DDT was outlawed in the U.S. in 1972, its residues persist in our environment and in our bodies. Almost all of us alive today will carry residues of DDT derivatives, such as DDE (a metabolite of DDT that is stored by the body), with us for the rest of our lives. And American manufacturers continue to make DDT and export it to developing nations (nearly 600,000 pounds of DDT were shipped between 1992 and 1994), where it contaminates their waters, animals, and food, and returns to us in crops exported back to the U.S.

Other pesticides with extensive use have been linked to hormone disruption. Atrazine, the most frequently used pesticide in the world, is a known endocrine disrupter and has been associated with increased numbers of mammary tumors, uterine cancer, and other cancers in animal studies (National Institute of Cancer at the National Institutes of Health). According to the EPA, in 1995 atrazine was the most widely used pesticide in U.S. agriculture, about 70 million pounds. The largest share of atrazine in our diet comes from milk, corn, sugar, and meat.

Nerve Toxins

For the past thirty years, pesticide exposure has been linked to neurotoxic effects in insects and in humans. High accident rates among pesticide workers and crop-dusters first suggested that these chemicals might have effects on the human nervous system, as they do on those of insects. More recently, broad-based studies associate pesticide exposure with damage to the nervous system and the brain, and for this reason the EPA has labeled an entire class of pesticides as Nerve Toxins (Category II).

Recent information on the Gulf War Syndrome, also linked to frequent and intense pesticide and chemical exposure, is providing additional insight into neurotoxic effects, which have included chronic fatigue, headaches, memory loss, and sleep disturbances. Similar symptoms have been experienced by farm and veterinary workers exposed to organophosphate insecticides. Psychological dysfunctions, mild paralysis, muscle cramps, and digestive problems are also associated with exposure to these insecticidal toxins.

A number of food additives and artificial food colorings found in prepared foods are considered nerve toxins by many researchers. The molecules of these chemicals can interfere with the chemical and electrical functioning of our brains, and it takes very little of the offending chemical to produce a toxic effect. In lab studies, the artificial sweetener aspartame has been linked to seizures, hydrolyzed vegetable protein to demonstrated brain-damaging properties, and MSG (monosodium glutamate) to brain tumors and brain lesions in lab animals. Additives such as MSG are termed "excito-toxins," so even if they do not cause nervous system damage, their chemical effect can overstimulate mental activity.

Heavy metals, particularly lead and mercury (and also cadmium), have been known as nerve toxins for hundred of years and are now found in much of our seafood. In recent testing of ocean tuna, all samples tested contained mercury. Aluminum has been associated with Alzheimer's disease in a number of research studies and appears not only as an environmental pollutant, but also as an intentional additive. Arsenic is also found as an unintentional pollutant in seafood and in some drinking water supplies.

Acute versus Chronic Exposure to Pesticides

An acute exposure is defined as *one exposure to a higher than safe amount or several exposures over a short period, usually by someone applying pesticides.* More than 123,000 cases of pesticide poisoning were reported to American poison control centers in 1995. Although very few deaths occurred, in California alone about 1,500 illnesses from occupational pesticide exposure are reported to doctors each year, and about 3,000 are estimated to occur. An entire category of pesticides is specifically labeled by the EPA as poison, meaning extremely high acute toxicity or "Category I" chemicals. But manuals written for physicians indicate that acute exposures to all classes of pesticides can be highly toxic, potentially causing convulsions and death. The World Health Organization (WHO) estimates that worldwide, more than two million cases of pesticide exposure occur annually with possibly 220,000 deaths. But some researchers estimate as many as 25 million cases of pesticide exposure occur each year.

Chronic exposure is defined as *mild, persistent low-level exposure.* California school children recently reported mild symptoms of nausea and respiratory problems following an accidental airborne exposure to pesticides at their school, located next to agricultural fields. In California alone, 758 schools have been identified where potential exposure could occur to the pesticide methyl bromide. This is a highly toxic fumigant with a restricted-use rating by the EPA, identified as a developmental toxin. More than 17 million pounds were used in California agriculture in 1995. Sadly, its heaviest application is on foods frequently eaten by children, such as grapes and strawberries.

Chemical Exposure and Chronic Health Problems

Exposure to pesticides, chemicals in meats, heavy metals in fish, unintentional pollutants, and the more toxic food additives should be avoided, especially when we are already ill. Patients with cancer, Alzheimer's disease, AIDS or suppressed immune systems, and heart disease should be especially careful in their selection of foods (National Academy of Sciences, 1993). Chemical exposure has also been linked to autoimmune conditions, in which the body turns its defenses against itself in a confused response.

Chemical sensitivity, which involves an overly reactive or allergic response to environmental chemicals, has become more prevalent in modern industrial societies. People with chemical sensitivity or autoimmune disorders may experience symptoms after eating chemically treated produce or products, or in some cases, just from being around the produce or the packing material. Soaking produce in bleach or washing it with detergent still may not remove enough spray residue to be tolerated.

An essential element in recovery from chemical sensitivity can be a diet of food grown naturally in healthy soil without synthetic chemicals or other contaminating processes—in other words, a completely organic and chemical-free diet.

Long-term or Latent Effects of Chemical Exposure

Nearly half of all nonorganic produce and grains contain legal levels of pesticide residues (FDA–1995). Little research is available to indicate the long-term effects of chemicals, even these commonly used pesticides, on the average person. Unfortunately, the studies on animals typically last only six months. Extended studies generally last no more than two years. None of the research designs can duplicate the daily effects of a lifetime of exposure. However, the data from the agricultural industry on cancer rates among farmworkers suggests genuine cause for concern. In an occupation with healthier than normal profiles, incidence of a dozen kinds of cancer and leukemia are definitely higher than in the general population.

Impact on Wildlife

In recent times, animals ranging from alligators in Florida to polar bears in Alaska have failed to reproduce, or have produced offspring with birth defects or serious health conditions. Scientist believe that birds of prey, fish, amphibians, and other wildlife are being exposed to estrogen-altering pesticides and other chemicals. In areas where oil spills have occurred, fish, birds, and even insects have been slow to return or have not returned at all.

The chemicals become more concentrated as they progress through the food chain. Eagles and other large birds that eat insects and rodents contaminated with persisting DDT acquire huge amounts of that chemical that are sometimes fatal; this was a common occurrence in the 1960s and was one of the main reasons DDT was banned. Similarly, in lakes and rivers, when large fish eat the small, contaminated fish, the toxic burden is passed along. High concentrations of chemicals can have serious consequences for humans as well.

These effects on wildlife foretell the danger to us all! Just as canaries were used to signal miners when the air became too dangerous to breathe, so the effects of pesticides on wildlife indicate the potential threat to human health. And damage can be caused by extremely small quantities of chemicals, particularly if the exposure occurs at the critical time of conception or development of new life.

Damage to the Environment

Pesticides and toxic chemicals can have harmful effects beyond the contamination of the air, water, and soil. Methyl bromide, for example, is classified as an ozone-destroying chemical under the national Clean Air Act. The World Health Organization has stated that the use of this chemical is responsible for up to 10% of ozone destruction worldwide.

The economic impact of toxic chemicals on the environment is estimated to be more than $8 billion annually. Researchers based the costs on: demands on public health ($787 million); cost of government attempts to prevent damage ($200 million); bird losses ($2 billion); and other factors relating to agricultural production (*BioScience*, 1992).

Adverse Effects on Agriculture

The downside of chemical use for agriculture includes groundwater contamination (costing nearly $2 billion); costs due to pesticide resistance ($1.4 billion); crop losses ($942 million); loss of natural pest predators and therefore natural pest control ($520 million); honeybee and pollination losses ($320 million); domestic animal deaths and contamination ($30 million); and fishery losses ($24 million) (*BioScience*, 1992). Although chemicals make agribusiness possible on a grand scale, the negative effects are enormous: degenerative disease in farmers and their families, the contamination of the land, air, and water, and the risk of damaging our farmland and environment beyond repair.

Agricultural Toxins: The Bottom Line

There are many instances in which profits speak louder than people, when it seems that the health of our planet, and the creatures who inhabit it, are valued less than the bottom line. It certainly appears that way in agriculture where the sale of chemicals to farmers is big business. Farmers spray their fields with thousands of different herbicides, insecticides, and other pesticides, and treat their produce with fungicides and fumigants for protection during shipping. In truth, few of the scientists, manufacturers, and farmers are fully aware of the consequences of their actions. Many of these chemicals kill natural pests and their predators, throwing off the ecological balance of Nature. The result is that even more potent chemicals are needed to eradicate the pests, which develop a resistance to previously used chemicals.

HOW TO DEAL WITH FOOD POLLUTION

I am a big supporter of the natural and organic food movements. I know that both manufacturers and consumers value the modern industrialized method of food production, but I favor minimizing crop spraying, food processing, and the use of food additives. In many cases, processed food provides the incentive for the manufacture and sale of chemical products. Fortunately, many food chemicals are safe, and more research funding is allocated to food additives than to any other area of industrial chemical use. However, the huge amount of agricultural and food processing chemicals utilized annually obviously interferes with potential life on our planet.

Safeguards and Concerns: *The good news and the bad news*

<u>The Good News:</u> We are fortunate to have a national food safety program. A century ago there was no government regulation of food additives and no monitoring of food safety. When our grandparents bought patent medicines, they could have gotten literally anything! Food and drug safety was still in its infancy. Foods were preserved by storing them on a block of ice, in the "ice box." Botulism and salmonella were rampant, and it was not unusual to hear about a family member who perished after a Sunday picnic dinner.

With the growth of cities, the mass marketing of food, and the development of agribusiness, it has been essential to have national safety standards and the monitoring of our food supply. Within the federal government, it is the EPA that sets the tolerance levels for the amounts of pesticide residues allowable in foods. The EPA also analyzes the levels of pollution in the air and in ground and surface water. However, this analysis occurs after the fact of the pollution.

The Food and Drug Administration (FDA) tests at random to determine whether pesticide residues on food fall within the legal limits. The FDA also registers and monitors additives in processed foods. It sets the legal limits for drug residues in meat, milk, eggs, and poultry, and standardizes nutritional information and food labeling. The USDA (U.S. Department of Agriculture) is responsible for food hygiene and safety standards for both domestic and imported foods and the inspection of all food-processing and meat-packing plants. Each of these agencies are typically overworked, understaffed, and underfunded, given the scale of their responsibility. So, consumer awareness is crucial to our individual protection from problems with chemical exposure.

The Bad News: When it comes to the safety of pesticides and chemical residues, the burden of proof is on the manufacturer, but they don't always follow through by providing the research necessary to assure safety. In California, for example, voters mandated that the most hazardous pesticides be tested. But eleven years later, that testing still has not been done, despite the ongoing exposure of school children to airborne pesticides such as methyl bromide, and the yearly contamination of California foods with more than 72 million pounds of agricultural pesticides (1995 figure from the California Department of Agriculture).

In reality, everyone who touches food is responsible for consumer safety—the farmer, picker, shipper, manufacturer, grocery store, and cook. Chemical additive manufacturers are responsible for proving that a new additive is safe for human consumption. However, since these are never tested on humans (or are they?), consumers cannot really depend on their safety. Once it goes to market, it is up to each of us to support or not support specific products. With our consumer dollars, we not only approve the practices of growers, producers, and manufacturers, we also reward them. Making informed food choices among the products that are available to us is the source of our greatest power to influence our personal health and that of our family.

The last word is not in on the long-term effects of food and environmental chemical interactions. As we stated earlier, research has proven that even individual chemicals that are nontoxic alone may present a risk when combined with other chemicals.

When we eat highly chemicalized foods, we take a risk. The health of our planet is also at stake. Overall, I believe that we should do everything in our personal power to avoid or minimize the use of chemicals and processed foods. Eating wholesome, natural, and organic foods, especially those grown locally and eaten fresh, offers long-range benefits for the health of our bodies and our environment.

HOW TO PROTECT YOURSELF FROM FOOD POLLUTION

1. **Minimize your intake of processed foods** and foods likely to have pesticide residues. This will reduce chemical insults and potential problems before they occur.

2. **Eat more fruits and vegetables** that are high in antioxidants, such as vitamin A and beta-carotene, vitamins C and E, zinc, and selenium. Also, take supplemental antioxidants.

3. **Gradually give up or minimize using refined sugar, caffeine, alcohol, and nicotine** to reduce the chemical burden on the body, and especially on the liver. For more information and specific guidance on this important process, which offers the beginning of real healing for many people, see my book, *The Detox Diet: The How-To and When-To Guide for Cleansing the Body.*

4. **Eat organically grown foods whenever possible.**

5. **Support the organizations that are your advocates,** including the Environmental Working Group, Mothers and Others, the National Campaign for Pesticide Reform, the National Coalition Against the Misuse of Pesticides (NCAMP), the Natural Resources Defense Council, and the Pesticide Action Network of North America (PANNA).

6. **Stay informed.** Read books that provide in-depth information, such as *Our Stolen Future, Diet for a Poisoned Planet, Living Downstream, Designer Poisons,* and *Toxic Deception.*

7. **Visit Web sites** with the latest updates, such as the Environmental Working Group at www.ewg.org and the Pesticide Action Network—PANNA at www.panna.org/panna/.

8. **Maintain an optimistic attitude.** An otherwise healthy lifestyle of exercise, stress management, and good dietary habits will reduce the risks that chemicals pose to your health.

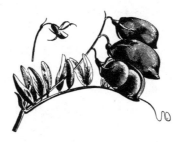

CHAPTER THREE

Pesticides and Pollution in Our Food Chain

◆

Chemical toxins can enter our food at any stage in its growing or processing cycle. They may be added to the soil before or during planting, or sprayed on fields; they may be used at the harvest, or during shipping and storage. Contaminants can be introduced through air, water, and soil, as well as through the byproducts of food cultivation such as pesticides, toxins in fertilizer, and accidental pollution, as well as chemicals used in building, at home, and in landscaping.

HOW DANGEROUS ARE PESTICIDES TO OUR HEALTH?

The effects of direct and repeated pesticide exposure can be seen in the accounts of a toxic spill of metam sodium that occurred in northern California in 1991. Metam sodium is a gas used mainly for soil fumigation before cultivation, so toxic that fields cannot be planted for several weeks after it is applied. In 1991, a railroad accident spilled 20,000 gallons of this chemical into the Sacramento River, killing all aquatic life for a 45-mile stretch of the river, as well as bald eagles and falcons who ate the fish, plus local deer, raccoons, bats, and other wildlife. Initially, several hundred people in the area were hospitalized with immediate health problems, including rashes, headaches, dizziness, and irritations involving the eyes, skin, and the respiratory and digestive tracts. Two years later, more than 700 residents of a town downstream continued to experience illness, primarily chemical sensitivity, arthritis, asthma, and chronic fatigue, for some so extreme that even walking was difficult. Of the eleven women who were pregnant at the time, five suffered miscarriages, a rate of 45%.

On California farms, metam sodium is used most often as a fumigant in raising carrots, potatoes, and tomatoes. Although the EPA has identified it as a potentially cancer-causing chemical, the California Department of Agriculture records that more than 15 million pounds were used just in California in 1995, more than three times the amount used in 1991 when the spill occurred.

A Brief History of Chemical Pesticides

The common ancestor of all modern toxic pesticides was the organophosphate, DEFP (diethylfluorophosphate), which was synthesized in Germany in 1932 as a byproduct of the research to develop nerve gas. Although DEFP is different in structure, it is related to the nerve poisons used in World War II. DDT, another organophosphate developed at the same time, was used successfully to control typhus in Italy and mosquito-borne diseases in tropical areas. When chemical insecticides were introduced in the U.S. following the war in the late 1940s, they helped increase crop yields dramatically.

It wasn't until the 1960s that we became aware that pesticide use had a cost. Concerns were raised about potential health risks, environmental contamination, and the impact on wildlife after the release of the ground-breaking book, *Silent Spring* by Rachel Carson, who died of breast cancer. In the 1980s and 1990s, some emphasis has been placed on biological, cultural, and alternative methods of pest control, usually called integrated pest management (IPM). IPM includes a number of different strategies against pests, such as biological controls (helpful insects) and the use of less toxic insecticides. But despite such efforts, pesticide use continues to rise steadily. From 1993 to 1994, pesticide use increased by about 11% and then leveled off in 1995. The agriculture industry in the U.S. spent more than $7 billion on pesticides in 1994 and almost $8 billion in 1995.

Currently, more than 21,000 pesticides with 867 active ingredients (1996 figures) are registered for use. *Nationwide, more than three pounds of pesticides are used annually for every man, woman, and child; in California, that amount is more than double at 6.5 pounds per person.*

What Are Pesticides and How Do They Get Into Our Food?

The FDA describes a pesticide as "any substance intended to control, destroy, repel, or attract a pest." Any living organism that causes damage or economic loss or that transmits or produces disease may be targeted. Pests can be animals (like insects or mice), unwanted plants (such as weeds), or microorganisms (typically viruses and fungus) that interfere with agricultural goals.

Pesticides are used because they are toxic to pest life; unfortunately, they are also toxic to wildlife and people, and to the Earth.

For the past 20 years, the United States agricultural industry has used about a billion pounds of pesticides each year. Our country also ships these agricultural toxins around the world. Between 1992 and 1994, U.S. companies exported more than 110,000 tons of pesticides, many of them now illegal in our own country, primarily to developing nations (*Audubon*, 1/97). This included approximately 600,000 pounds of DDT. The pesticides come back to us in the foods we import—about a fourth of our national food supply; this is termed "the circle of poison."

We bring many of these chemicals (pesticides and pollutants) home with us in the products we buy at the supermarket. When the USDA recently performed a spot check of produce, they found that 71% of the foods sampled contained at least one pesticide residue. Almost all the samples were within the EPA tolerance, which means that it is legally acceptable for us to consume pesticides in the majority of our food. And since there are no labeling requirements for pesticides, most of us are unknowingly consuming a variety of them each day.

There is an overwhelming amount of research that links pesticide exposure to increased health risk. The National Library of Medicine lists more than 63,000 articles from medical journals on pesticides; there are more than 4,400 studies devoted to their adverse effects. The risks appear to be greatest for those who work with pesticides and for children in households where pesticides are used in the home or garden. Consumers are generally more concerned about the effects of traces of pesticides in foods, rather than the impact of direct exposure. Pesticides and other pollutants in our foods contribute to the toxic load on our bodies and the increased risk of neurotoxic diseases and cancer. Although there are no long-range studies to indicate whether *traces* of these chemicals that we are exposed to over time are really safe or not, most of us wonder.

Imported produce is often more dangerous because it may contain pesticide residues that have been determined by our government to be unsafe and therefore, have been made illegal. Recent findings showed that about half of the residues detected in imported items, such as bulb onions, apple juice, and green peas, were illegal. Illegal residues were also found on about one fourth of the imported pineapples, pears, and carrots. Other popular imported produce averaged 10% to 15% illegal residues compared with about 3% found on domestic produce (FDA 1992 and 1993, analyzed by the Environmental Working Group).

Are Very Small Traces of Pesticides in Our Foods Really That Risky?

The government currently allows pesticides and additives in food based on a policy of **relative risk**. Risk is determined by posing the *theoretical* question "How much of a given pesticide can be consumed that will only cause cancer in one person in a million?" Recently, tolerances have been increased to a theoretical cancer risk factor of two in a million. Estimates such as two in a million are clearly very abstract when you consider that current statistics suggest that, for all cancers combined from all causes, *one American in three will develop cancer in their lifetime.*

Sadly, pesticide tolerances are often based on the perceived needs of the agricultural industry (and chemical companies), rather than on safe levels of exposure, which may be much lower. Dr. Richard Jackson is a pediatrician with the California State Department of Health Services and co-author of the National Academy of Sciences' study entitled "Pesticides in the Diets of Infants and Children" (1993). In this report, he compares current pesticide tolerances to "setting the speed limit at 7,000 miles per hour and congratulating yourself that no one exceeds it. The tolerances are so high that clearly there's very little food out there that breaks the law."

What Do Scientists Know About the Long-Term Effects of Pesticides?

The 1996 hearings before the House of Representatives on the Gulf War Syndrome reveal the problems in assessing chemical exposure. Although some military personnel experienced symptoms immediately following their exposure to pesticides and chemicals, the results of their medical tests were normal for several years. It wasn't until six years after their initial exposure that major symptoms developed. At that point, physicians from the Veterans Administration indicated that there were no tests to identify a past chemical exposure or the cause of their problems.

Information on the health of farmers and farmworkers is even more revealing. Although this group of workers is generally healthier than people in most occupations (nonsmokers, physically active), it has had unusually high rates of cancer. A nine-year study in Wisconsin found that young farmers had cancerous lymphoma at rates three to six times higher than normal. In a ten-year study nationwide, agricultural extension workers (advisors who provide technical assistance to farmers) showed unusually high rates of leukemia (National Institutes of Health). Farmworkers and other occupations that work with pesticides have excessive rates of a number of cancers, including cancers of the brain, lip, lung, prostate, stomach, and testes, as well as melanoma and other skin cancers (Source: *Human Health Effects of Pesticides* by M. C. Keifer, Ed., Hanley & Belfus, Inc.: Philadelphia, 1997). Other studies that looked at health patterns among large numbers of workers found elevated rates of cancer of the pancreas, liver, and breast among farmworkers. They also have been shown to have higher rates of soft tissue sarcoma, Hodgkin's disease, non-Hodgkin's lymphoma, multiple myelomas, and leukemia.

PESTICIDES CLASSIFIED BY USE

Herbicides

Herbicides are used on the soil in the pre-planting period and in the early stages of cultivation to kill weeds, so that there will be less growth competition and easier harvesting. They are used more than any other type of pesticide; in 1995, over 755 million pounds of herbicides were produced in the United States, compared to 378 million pounds of insecticides and 109 million pounds of fungicides (USDA). Most of the herbicides are fairly toxic and potentially carcinogenic, such as the chemical 2,4-D. Their restricted-use ratings mean that they are meant to be applied only before planting or in areas where food crops won't be grown. Because herbicides are labor savers, they're used extensively. (This class of chemicals is discussed further on page 37.)

Insecticides

Insecticides are applied primarily during actual food cultivation to prevent insects from eating or otherwise damaging the crop. Plants absorb these chemicals, as well as minerals from the soil, while they are growing. Pesticide sprays are also used during harvesting. Some of these chemicals leach through the soil into the water table far below the surface, and cycle back into the soil, the plants, and the water used for irrigation.

> ## TYPES OF PESTICIDES CURRENTLY IN USE
>
> Pesticides can be grouped into several categories:
>
> *By use:*
> - **Herbicides**—used to kill weeds, usually prior to growing
> - **Insecticides**—used to kill insects and pests during the growing period
> - **Fungicides**—applied to retard molds and fungus
> - **Fumigants**—for controlling insects and damage during shipping and storage
>
> *By chemical structure:*
> - **Heavy and toxic metals**—such as mercury, cadmium, arsenic, and copper
> - **Organochlorides**—very strong chlorinated hydrocarbons that persist in the soil and our bodies
> - **Organophosphates and carbamates**—essentially nerve gases, these are shorter lived and include malathione, parathione, and carbaryl
> - **Triazines and other herbicides**—toxins designed to kill plants, which must be stronger than those used for insects; these include agent orange, paraquat, and the triazine family, such as atrazine

Neither the Earth nor our bodies can break down many of the synthetic chemicals used as insecticides. Therefore, they accumulate and remain in the soil and in our tissues. Some pesticides begin to break down within a few days, and most within weeks. Others remain in the environment for two to three years. There are also chemicals, such as DDT, that remain for decades, and at this point, researchers suggest that every person on Earth has some DDT in their body tissues. Since 1 to 2 billion pounds of pesticides have been used every year in the United States for the past 20 years, the burden of accumulating toxins on the land and on our bodies is definitely growing.

Fungicides are mainly sprayed on harvested food to prevent mold and tend to have lower toxicity to mammals. But even in this class of pesticide, toxicity varies widely from elementary sulfur (with no known cumulative effect) to mercury compounds (which are highly toxic, accumulate, and can cause severe illness in a single dose).

Some fungicides have been associated with cancer, birth defects, and thyroid problems. Captan, for example, is proven to cause genetic changes (mutagenic) and cancer in animals and is regulated as a possible cancer-causing (carcinogenic) agent in humans.

Fumigants are frequently used on fruits, vegetables, and grains in preparation for shipping or storage to inhibit destruction by molds or bugs, or to retard premature sprouting. This type of pesticide poses a threat because of the high concentrations of chemicals that are still on the foods when they reach the consumer. Fumigants are also of concern to workers using them, because the airborne gases are inhaled. Since many of these chemicals are derived from solvents or from oil-based products, they tend to persist in the environment for at least several months.

Much of the produce that we buy in the supermarket has been directly treated with pesticides after it is fully grown or harvested. For example, fruits, especially dried fruits such as dates and figs, are often fumigated with chemicals such as methyl bromide to protect them from insects and molds. Such pesticides can trigger irritations, allergies, or symptoms of asthma. Many grains and legumes, particularly wheat, rice, and corn, are also fumigated periodically during storage. In a recent review of pesticide residues, 91% of the wheat sampled contained pesticide residues. It has been suggested that some forms of wheat allergy, which have been associated with learning problems, may actually be a reaction to the neurotoxic effects of the high chemical residues on the grain, particularly on nonorganic whole wheat.

Spraying with pesticides to keep insects away during shipping is common for imported fruits such as papayas, mangoes, and pineapples. Bananas are less likely to be sprayed, but are often gassed or fumigated with ethylene before they are shipped to help them ripen.

Unfortunately, the EPA frequently finds that a pesticide is unsafe *after* it has been in use for years. For example, DBCP (dibromo-chloropropane), which was sprayed on Hawaiian pineapples for decades and contaminated the waters there, was banned in 1979 because of its toxicity, but it will remain in the environment into the new millennium.

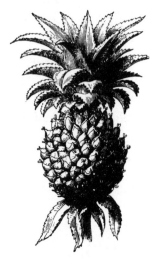

PESTICIDES CLASSIFIED BY THEIR CHEMICAL STRUCTURE

Heavy and Toxic Metals

Many common pesticides incorporate metals with chemicals. Some of these metals are now illegal, such as thallium-based products, banned in 1968. Examples of pesticides in this class currently in use include arsenic and chromic acid (from chromium), both herbicides used in wood treatments, and both known cancer-causing agents classified with the most toxic rating of Category I highly acute toxicity.

Organochlorides

This is a toxic class of chemicals that destroys pests by attacking their central nervous system. Many of the pesticides in this class, including DDT, are now illegal in the U.S. because they do not break down, so their toxic effects tend to remain over time.

Organochlorides accumulate in the environment and in our bodies, particularly in fatty tissue, and these chemicals can last for a lifetime. They have been linked to numerous degenerative conditions including cancer, reproductive and developmental problems, birth defects, genetic damage, and neurotoxic effects. In animal studies, organochlorides have also been shown to cause birth defects and genetic changes.

Researchers from the National Cancer Institute (NIH) confirm that people in the U.S. may be exposed to organochlorides through the contamination of imported foods. This process has been referred to by some as the "circle of poison."

Because of their acknowledged toxicity in humans and animals, three of the most commonly used organochlorides were banned—DDT in 1972, Aldrin in 1974, and Endrin in 1979. These poisons and their relatives still remain in the soil after many years of spraying, but they no longer kill the pests, just the people, birds, and animals that consumed the contaminated food, water, or insects containing these toxic compounds. And DDT for example, can be stored in the human body for decades, often as DDE, which is linked to increased cancer incidence. Toxaphene, an organochloride still in use, is identified by the EPA as a probable human carcinogen; like DDT, it is neurotoxic and an endocrine-disrupting pesticide and labeled by the EPA as a highly acute toxin.

Organophosphates

These are the most common pesticides used today, with malathione and parathione leading the group. Although they break down into less harmful chemicals within weeks of their use, initially they are more toxic than the earlier organochlorides and have been linked to numerous cases of fatal poisoning among farmworkers. Organophosphates also operate by interfering with nerve conduction and can lead to convulsions and death when they are inhaled, ingested, or absorbed through the skin in large quantities.

When trace amounts of organophosphate pesticides are consumed regularly in foods, they may have a genetic effect that could generate cancer or birth defects, and they may be toxic to the nervous system and brain. Of the most frequently used organophosphates, mevinphos and parathion are labeled as Category I acute toxins (EPA), and malathion and parathion are also identified as endocrine-disrupters that can cause cancer. The Environmental Working Group reports that every day, about 77,000 American infants are exposed to unsafe levels of organophosphates in fresh produce and in baby food preparations such as apple juice, applesauce, pears, and peaches.

Carbamates

The carbamate class of pesticides is also widely used today. Like organochlorides and the organophosphates, they interfere with the function of the nervous system. Although they can be highly toxic, spontaneous recovery is more often possible when workers are exposed to carbamate pesticides. Unlike DDT and related chemicals, carbamates pass through the body fairly rapidly; no evidence has been found that they are stored in the body (chemical bioaccumulation). However, these pesticides are also suspected of causing birth defects. Of carbamates currently in use, aldicarb, carbaryl, and methomyl have been identified as endocrine disrupters and are labeled for restricted use only. Carbaryl is also categorized by the EPA as a nerve toxin. Aldicarb, carbofuran, methomyl, and oxamyl are all considered Category I acute toxins.

Triazines

These are one of the most widely used classes of herbicides in the world. Of these, atrazine (an endocrine-disrupter) is used more than any pesticide in the U.S. and for the past ten years, at least 70 million pounds of atrazine have been applied annually. Other extensively used triazines include cyanazine (a developmental toxin) and simazine (restricted use category). One of the greatest dangers of herbicides is that the runoff contaminates groundwater and reservoirs, finding its way into drinking water. A 1994 study of tests on tap and drinking waters found that more than 14 million people routinely drink water contaminated with these chemicals (EWG).

Other Herbicides

Researchers have noted that chemicals used to kill plants tend to be even stronger than those that destroy insects. Well known examples include Agent Orange (used to defoliate the forests of Vietnam) and paraquat (used on marijuana fields here in the States). Both of these herbicides are reported to cause serious reproductive damage.

Use of herbicides such as diuron, molinate, paraquat, and simazine have each averaged close to a million pounds annually in California for the past five years. Because they're used in such great quantities on non-food crops (such as cotton), along highways, and over forests, they not only contaminate farmland, and surface and groundwater, they pose a significant health risk.

How Are Pesticides Monitored?

Created in 1970, the Environmental Protection Agency (EPA) is responsible for regulating the use, distribution, and disposal of pesticides. The EPA approves and registers pesticides, reviews the testing on their safety, and evaluates each chemical against legal standards for human health, the environment, and wildlife. The Food and Drug Administration (FDA) monitors pesticide residues on food to determine if the amount falls within the legal guidelines. Given the enormous scope of their task and the high economic stakes for pesticide manufacturers and food growers, it is understandable that this is a difficult industry to monitor.

The state of California is an interesting example of how even the most progressive policies concerning pesticide monitoring cannot match the economic clout of agribusiness. The state has its own registry and monitoring program, one of the strictest in the country. And the state university system, the University of California, has an excellent research program in integrated pest management, one of the best alternatives we have to the use of pesticides. Yet because of its huge growing

COMMON MISCONCEPTIONS ABOUT PESTICIDES

1. *Pesticides are considered safe for use as long as they are not actually used during the growth phase of the plant*: This statement ignores the general effects of using pesticides before planting, in non-growing areas around farms, after harvest, or during shipping. These multiple and extensive uses of pesticides at times other than when the plant is growing increase the toxic burden on the land, air, water and on human and animal life.

   Costs to the environment do not appear to motivate growers to decrease chemical use. Residues remain in the soil and wash into our lakes and rivers where they contaminate drinking water and aquatic life. They seep through the Earth into the water table—our precious ground water—the source of all springs and deep wells. Residues in the soil cling to the crops planted next in that soil, saturate root vegetables, and destroy insects that normally play a healthy role in agriculture.

2. *"Natural" pesticides are better than manufactured ones*: We put a high value on things that are labeled as "natural." However, when it comes to pesticides, natural poisons can be just as toxic as synthetics. The World Health Organization (WHO) points out that many of the most highly poisonous materials known are of natural origin. The lethal poison strychnine is a good example. *Plant-based pesticides* with a toxic rating that are currently in use include three insecticides derived from pyrethrums, all endocrine-disrupters: cypermethrin, fenvalerate, and permethrin. In California agriculture alone, over 400,000 pounds of permethrin was used in 1995. WHO calls for more thorough testing of all biological agents.

3. *Nerve toxins (organochlorides, organophosphates, and carbamates) that are deadly to insects aren't that harmful to humans*: Research and medical case studies have shown that most pesticides are toxic to the nervous systems of insects and of people. How can we believe that they have no effect on us? Research has not yet sufficiently explored the possible link between the presence of neurotoxic chemicals in over half of our food supply and the dramatic increases in learning problems and hyperactivity in our children.

area, California continues to be an exceptionally heavy user of agricultural chemicals. Currently in California alone, more than 212 million tons of pesticides are dumped on fields and crops each year.

Although legislation mandated by California voters requires the identification and labeling of toxic pesticides, these new laws still have not decreased pesticide use. Over the past five years, the use of the most toxic pesticides in California has increased an astonishing 34%, up to 72 million pounds of pesticides with hazardous ratings (PANNA). This increase wasn't due to increased acreage; rather it was an increase in the intensity of pesticide use, expanding from 18 pounds per acre in 1991 to almost 25 pounds per acre by 1995. Crop by crop, this "war on bugs" has become intense; strawberries, for example, are treated with more than 300 pounds of pesticides for every acre grown.

The Good News About Pesticide Reduction: What We Do Can Make a Difference

Banning DDT may decrease breast cancer. In Israel, from 1976 to 1986, death rates due to breast cancer actually decreased by 8%—and among young women, rates decreased by 34%. It has been suggested that the banning of two organochloride pesticides (DDT and lindane) in 1978 could have contributed to the decrease. These pesticides were used extensively in dairy farming, and contaminant levels in milk were 5 to 10 times those in the United States. Within two years of the ban, DDE (from DDT) in cow's milk had decreased by 43% and lindane byproducts had dropped 98% (*Designer Poisons*).

Strawberry fields forever.... free of methyl bromide. Strawberries are the most contaminated of all food crops in the United States. In fact, 70% of the strawberry samples tested by the FDA in 1995 had chemical residues—of 30 different pesticides! Of these, methyl bromide is considered one of the most toxic. In 1993 and 1995, over 4 million pounds of methyl bromide were used on California strawberry fields.

But in Holland, strawberries have been grown on a large scale without methyl bromide for more than 10 years. Yields are typically higher than those of California, because organic growing practices make high-density plantings possible. Although it takes extra attention and work, it appears to be worth it.

The rise of the organic food industry is an American success story. Did you know that organic food production is the fastest growing sector in US agriculture? Annual sales are now $4 billion, and the organic food business has grown about 20% a year for the last seven years. These successes demonstrate that it is possible to create a thriving agricultural economy without the use of toxic chemicals (*Rising Toxic Tide*, PANNA). (See Chapter 7 on *Organics*.)

POLLUTION ON THE FARM

Our industrial economy marches on, oblivious to the toxic accumulation of 150 years of industrial practices. Our air, soil, and water appear to be universally contaminated, possibly beyond repair, although I wish not to believe it. There is hope if we can re-embrace Nature and natural methods of food cultivation and production.

Contamination from Fertilizers

Nitrogen-based fertilizers are commonly used to stimulate plant growth and create bigger crop yields. These fertilizers can create imbalances in the soil and cause depletion of other important trace minerals, such as chromium, selenium, iodine, and lithium. Trace mineral deficiencies are linked to a wide variety of symptoms and degenerative diseases. Nitrate contamination can create nitrosamines, a highly carcinogenic byproduct. Excessive nitrates from fertilizers wash into rivers and seep into the water table; they were found to pollute drinking water supplies in 40 states (EWG). In some areas, nitrates have literally poisoned the farm lands and water sources.

Fertilizer may also contain hazardous recycled industrial waste. From 1990 to 1995, 270 million pounds of industrial waste was shipped to fertilizer manufacturers throughout the United States. Some of the waste contained heavy metals such as mercury and lead, as well as dioxin residues (EWG). When the fertilizer was shipped to farmers, there was no labeling or other indication of the recycled industrial content. This recycled material further contaminates the soil and enters our food chain. The chemicals also accumulate in run-off waters and end up in underground aquifers where groundwater is stored, or in lakes and rivers.

The use of chemical fertilizers and toxic pesticides can damage or kill the naturally occurring organisms in the soil, such as nitrogen-fixing bacteria, that helps plants grow by generating nitrogen. It can also destroy creatures that are beneficial to agriculture, such as birds, bees, and earthworms. As a result, the physical quality of the soil can deteriorate, due to compacting, reduced water retention, and poor soil aeration. All these effects brought on by chemical fertilizers decrease the nutrient content of crops and make them more vulnerable to disease (NCAMP).

Water Pollution

The USDA estimates that 50 million people in the US get their drinking water from ground water that is potentially contaminated by pesticides and other agricultural chemicals. A 1995 survey of tap water found herbicides in the tap water of 28 out of 29 midwestern cities, some at levels that exceeded the EPA Lifetime Health Advisory Level (EWG). Another study found one or more pesticides in the water of two thirds of the cities and 10% of the rural communities tested.

The main sources of water contamination include:

• *Chemical plants, pulp mills, steel factories, and other industries* dumped more than a billion pounds of toxic chemicals into America's rivers, lakes, and coastal waters between 1990 and 1994, including phosphoric acid, ammonia, and sulfuric acid. Some particularly toxic chemicals found in groundwater include DDT, vinyl chloride, methylene chloride, carbon tetrachloride, TCE (trichloroethylene), benzene, xylenes, chemical pesticides, and petroleum byproducts.

   Millions of pounds of toxic metals were also dumped (EWG). This waste is polluting underground water—the groundwater that feeds into springs, lakes, and streams, provides irrigation, and supplies wells. Federal warnings in 1997 indicated that fish from more than 1,660 American waterways were so contaminated with mercury that they should not be eaten (EWG).

   Areas near waste sites also contain PCBs and metals such as lead and mercury. A survey conducted ten years ago found 46 pesticides in the groundwater of at least 26 states.

   Current estimates suggest that between 30% and 50% of our groundwater is contaminated, which may be irreversible. It is estimated that it would take billions of dollars to even begin to clean up our water resources, rivers, and lakes, and we haven't fully developed the technology needed for restoration on such a massive scale.

• *Agricultural activities.* The levels of herbicides such as atrazine and simazine exceed the new cancer risk benchmark for tap water in 245 communities in agricultural states. These toxins also contaminate the tap water of 374 Midwestern towns (EWG). In Ohio, in more than 100 communities, at least five different herbicides were found in the tap water.

Many agricultural practices associated with raising animals are also known to contaminate groundwater and rivers: in North Carolina, rivers have been contaminated with nitrates from hog production; and the Chesapeake Bay in Maryland has been polluted with nitrates from chicken farming. In California, the contamination of wetlands with agricultural drainage water in the Central Valley became legendary when 42,000 acres of farmland ultimately lost their irrigation water due to selenium contamination, at an economic cost to the area of more than $67 million.

- *Mining and dispensing of radioactive materials and other waste.* Land disposal of metal, chemical, and radioactive wastes is an inefficient way of storing pollutants and always runs the risk of contaminating ground water; burying the problem is only a short-term solution. But it is less expensive than other more responsible solutions, and changing established ways of doing things is always an uphill battle.

- *Underground storage tanks.* Gasoline is the most common substance stored this way; leakage of tanks can contaminate water sources. Pesticides can persist in the groundwater long after their use has been discontinued. DBCP (dibromochloropane), a soil fumigant banned in California in 1977, is still found in groundwater twenty years later in quantities great enough to pose a significant health risk in agricultural areas.

- *Recreational vehicle pollution.* Gasoline and its additives, such as MTBE, add hazardous pollution to lakes and rivers. Laws are currently being drafted and enacted to deal with this issue.

Air Pollution

The general population can be exposed to agricultural pollution through drift from sprayed applications, overspray, or out-gassing of products in shipping or storage. Airborne pesticides are a particular problem for farm families and workers because chemicals also attach to dust particles and persist even when no contamination can be measured in the air. They also pose a threat for rural residents. As a case in point, air quality at a California school located next to strawberry acreage registered pollution levels 10 times the safe tolerance when the fields were pretreated with methyl bromide. Pollution from pesticide manufacturing can also be a problem. In Arkansas, 20% of the children living near an herbicide plant had residues of 2,4-D (endocrine-disrupter) in their urine.

Reducing Lead in Our Lifetime!

There are so few national examples of beating pollution that we have chosen one from the environmental arena to demonstrate how pollution can be reduced if we have the political will and industrial cooperation to do so. Lead had been pervading our water, homes, fish, and other foods for decades, and was a serious health risk, especially for children. But the number of young children with potentially harmful blood lead levels has dropped 85% over the last 20 years as a result of government efforts. Lead was banned from house paint in 1978. U.S. canners stopped using lead solder in 1991. And a 25-year phaseout of lead in gasoline reached its goal in 1995 (FDA). There is more to be done, because lead contamination still occurs in older homes and buildings from deteriorating paint. *But this 85% reduction is an example of what can be done if we set our minds and hearts to it and back it with dollars.*

What About Our Future?

It's a tall order, but contamination of our food supply and drinking water by pesticides and other pollutants is at a crisis point. We need to become better informed about this crucial issue and find ways to express our views, address this problem, and find solutions *now*! When more people realize that our health—and that of our planet—is more important than increased food production, fewer pests, and higher profits, we will have the power to influence both the food industry and our future health.

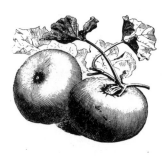

CHAPTER FOUR

Food Processing and Additives

◆

WHAT'S ADDED
AND WHAT TO AVOID

Why are chemicals used in our foods today? There was a time when wild foods were sought and gathered from a relatively unpolluted Earth. Cleaner oceans, lakes, and rivers were home to nutritious fish. Wild animals provided protein foods to hunters and their tribes. As the human population multiplied, farming and animal husbandry progressed, trade specialties developed, and village markets shared a variety of goods among a diversity of people. Techniques for food preparation and preservation, such as pickling, salting, and smoking, were developed to deal with the new problems of storage, waste, and foodborne illnesses. Today, with advanced technology, our modern food industry's reliance on processing and additives continues to increase. Is this evolution, or are we sacrificing our health for the sake of technological advances?

The food industry continues to create new chemicals with which to manipulate, preserve, and transform our food. Scientists are able to mimic natural flavors, color foods to make them look more "natural" or "fresh," preserve foods for longer and longer periods of time, and create altered versions of breads, crackers, fruits, vegetables, meats, dairy products and more. Now there are even "foods" that are made entirely from chemicals. Coffee creamers, sugar substitutes, and candies consist almost completely of artificial ingredients. This manipulation can have a profound effect on our body's unique biochemical balance.

Types of Food Additives

Food additives are typically classified by groups according to how they are used in processing. The following will provide you with a basic overview for understanding the complexities of the food industry, and offers a foundation for understanding and evaluating food labels. (For more detailed information on individual food additives, see the Appendix, or Chapter 11 in *Staying Healthy with Nutrition*.)

- **Sweeteners** are added to processed foods as flavor enhancers. They are the most common additive group and they are consumed in the largest volume (about 150 pounds for every person in the U.S. each year). Examples include sugar, fructose (extracted from fruit), corn syrup and corn sweetener, brown sugar, molasses, barley malt, beet sugar, and rice syrup. Excess intake has been associated with such problems as diabetes, hypoglycemia, depression, atherosclerosis, and heart disease.

  Stevia is a natural sweetener (an herbal extract) that also appears to have health benefits.

  <u>In general, it is wise to limit even natural sweeteners in the diet, and obtain sugars from foods.</u>

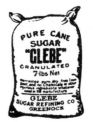

- **Artificial sweeteners** are chemical sweeteners. Currently, there are three (the fourth, cyclamate, is banned), with varied status:

  Aspartame is widely used, but controversial due to its role as an excitoxin to the brain and nervous system. As Nutrasweet or Equal, it is currently the most commonly used artificial sweetener.

  Saccharin has not been banned but remains on probationary status, possibly because of public demand.

  Ace K (acesulfame potassium) is being evaluated for approval. It is used on a very limited basis, although it is known to cause an increase in tumor production in animal studies.

  <u>I suggest avoiding all of these artificial sweeteners.</u>

- **Flavorings** are the largest group of all the additives with more than 2,000 different flavorings (500 natural and more than 1,500 synthetic). Flavor additives are used to attain a certain taste in foods that is consistent and uniform to meet the consumer's expectations.

WHY CHEMICALS ARE ADDED TO OUR FOODS

1. *To improve shelf life or storage time.* This was the original reason for using additives. The special "curing" of foods and the development of prepackaged (protected), processed foods were said to allow more food to get to more people and prevent waste and spoilage. Most canned foods are heat treated and vacuum packed so that they can be preserved and stored for years. Many fruits, especially dried fruits, are treated with sulfur dioxide or sprayed with chemicals to prevent their destruction by air, molds, or bugs. Many breads and baked goods are treated (or "embalmed") with chemicals to improve shelf life. Such methods may be helpful to the manufacturer, but not necessarily beneficial to the health and longevity of the consumer.

2. *To make food convenient and easy to prepare.* Separate dishes or entire meals boxed or frozen as TV dinners or microwaveable meals, as well as cake mixes and other ready-to-make foods, are examples of convenience foods. Modern techniques of food processing have created thousands of new products that allow consumers to save time and shelf life to be extended (sometimes indefinitely).

   Because families today are often comprised of a working single parent or two working parents, we seem to have less time to spend on food preparation. Manufacturers capitalize on this and prepare foods for us, packing them in flashy boxes, jars, or cans, freezing them, or making "instant" versions so that we can simply add water, heat, microwave, or otherwise prepare them with very little effort. But there is a cost for this effortless preparation—the food that remains after processing may retain very few nutrients and offer very little vitality. Instant mashed potatoes, breakfast cereals, instant oatmeal, cookies, hot dogs, luncheon meats, cups of noodles, frozen meals, and thousands of other products fit into this category.

3. *To increase nutritional value.* Many food products have synthetic vitamins added to them and are sold as "enriched" foods. They are of

moderate benefit to consumers. Ironically, these added vitamins are often the same ones that were removed during processing. The great flaw here, though, is that many important vitamins and minerals are processed out of whole foods and not fully added back into them. Vitamin B_6, chromium, and zinc are a few examples of important nutrients that are lost during the processing of grains and flours and not replaced. For that reason, it is better to eat whole grains. Occasionally, foods are "fortified," which means that they have an added nutrient that is not normally found in the original food. Cow's milk fortified with vitamin D is a common example.

4. *To improve the flavor of foods.* Many flavorings, both natural and artificial, are used in an attempt to create greater consumer appeal. Making foods sweeter, saltier, or spicier often tantalizes the taste buds and fosters a desire for the repeated use. The unique flavor of many processed and packaged foods is created through much time and expense on the part of the manufacturer. Salt and sugar are the two most common flavorings. Monosodium glutamate is another common "flavor enhancer."

5. *To enhance the attractiveness of food products and improve consumer acceptance.* This is a scary one, because the chemicals used to maintain or enhance a product's color or prevent it from being discolored are often the more potentially toxic substances. Even our "natural" produce, the fruits and vegetables, are exposed to such chemicals. Oranges are often dipped in dyes to enhance their color. Chickens may be treated with yellow dyes to keep their skin looking "healthy." Sprays are used on produce to prevent insects and microorganisms from moving in or consuming them before they reach the consumer. Bananas are gassed, many other fruits and vegetables are sprayed with fungicides, and breads have added mold inhibitors. Unfortunately, what increases the selling power of many items in the eyes of consumers may not benefit their health.

Natural flavors are concentrated extracts that include essential oils, various spices, and natural plant oil extracts (oleo-resins). Most of these are considered safer than the synthetic versions, (two exceptions are nutmeg, when used in excess, and safrole, the toxic oil from saffron).

"Artificial flavors," the synthetic versions of natural flavors, are made from a great number of chemicals, and many flavors are made from a blend of chemicals. FDA regulations do not require flavoring chemicals to be specified on labels. Some of them can be mildly toxic to the nervous system, the kidneys, or liver, but generally appear to be safe when used in small quantities. They are commonly used in soft drinks, chewing gum, candy, ice creams, baked goods, puddings, and other desserts.

Flavor enhancers are intended to bring out or improve flavor, and include salt (sodium chloride) which can cause hypertension if used in excess, and MSG (monosodium glutamate) a known excitotoxin to the brain and nervous system, which can cause headaches or palpitations.

These additives should be minimized, and most people should avoid MSG.

- **Coloring agents,** typically synthetic, are probably the additives of greatest concern. I suggest we avoid artificially colored foods as much as possible.

  Natural colors (from natural sources) which appear to be quite safe include carotene, caramel, annatto, beet red, saffron, paprika, grape extract, and fruit and vegetable juice extracts.

  Synthetic (Artificial) colors, including those made from petroleum and coal-tar products, can be toxic and can have adverse health effects. Many have not been fully tested and a dozen have been withdrawn because research revealed them to be toxic or potentially cancer-causing. Other harmful effects include allergic reactions, links with behavior problems, short attention span, hyperactivity in children, and liver stress from metabolizing these chemicals. The fact that labeling doesn't indicate the specific coloring agents (other than tartrazine, yellow #5) added to food is further cause for concern, because we have no way of knowing what is safe. For example, Orange B has been banned, but not for coloring orange skins!

- **Preservatives** are another group of additives that cause concern. The include about 100 different chemicals used to prevent spoilage. These are required to be listed on the labels:

Chemicals that prevent fat from oxidizing (antioxidants), used in many packaged and bottled foods including shortening and vegetable oils, and foods that contain them, such as cereals and crackers. These antioxidant additives include BHT, banned in England, and BHA, both considered mild carcinogens.

Mold inhibitors (antimycotics) are used in breads, baked goods, cheeses, syrups, and other foods. Some mold inhibitors are considered quite safe, such as sorbic acid. Others, such as sodium or calcium propionate, may have mildly adverse effects. A third category includes naturally occurring substances such as lactic acid, which most people tolerate well, but cause symptoms in those with a specific condition, in this case a dairy intolerance.

Sequestrants are substances that prevent physical or chemical changes in food and preserve its appearance. Commonly used in dairy products and salad dressings, these relatively benign additives include EDTA and various salts of sodium, potassium, or calcium, such as calcium chloride.

Common preservatives also include salt and sugar, which have health concerns when used in excess, which they commonly are. Sulfur dioxide is used to preserve dried fruits, such as apricots, raisins, and peaches, as well as corn and wine. Sulfur compounds are known to cause allergic reactions.

- **Acids, alkalis, buffers, and neutralizers** may or may not be listed on the label. Mineral salts and acids may be used to adjust the acid-alkaline balance in foods, to make dough rise, or to enhance flavor. Some mild natural acids are quite safe: citric acid (from citrus fruits), malic acid (from apples), and tartaric acid (from grapes). Alkalis are additives that make the food less acid, such as baking powder and baking soda used in crackers, cookies, and candies. Buffers and neutralizers also adjust the acidity (pH) of food. This category includes baking powders that contain aluminum and aluminum hydroxide in cocoa and aluminum carbonate in prepared foods. I recommend that people minimize their aluminum exposure because of its continued link to brain dysfunction and Alzheimer's disease.

- **Bleaching and maturing agents** are used in flour products and sometimes in cheeses. Some are used to bleach flour or other foods; others are used to condition dough. Most of these are listed on the label; their safety ranges from harmless to questionable. Examples include bleaching agents, such as benzoyl peroxide and chlorine dioxide, and dough conditioners, such as potassium bromate and mineral salts.

- **Moisture controls** are chemicals that help prevent foods from drying out or becoming too moist. For example, calcium silicate is added to table salt to prevent caking. <u>Propylene glycol, glycerin, and sorbitol are other examples that are generally considered to be safe.</u>

- **Activity controls** are chemical agents that either slows or accelerates the ripening or aging of foods. They are most often used on fresh fruits and vegetables, which are unlabeled. For example, enzymes such as amylase may be used to stimulate the fermentation of sugar in the course of food processing and is a naturally occurring substance. <u>On the other hand, additives such as maleic hydrazide, used to prevent the sprouting of potatoes and onions, is potentially toxic.</u>

- **Emulsifiers** help to blend oils with water-soluble liquids to maintain the consistency of products such as mayonnaise and salad dressings, as stabilizers and thickeners. <u>The range of safety here is wide, from healthful additives such as lecithin to polysorbate 80, known to cause cancer.</u>

- **Texturizers** are stabliziers and processing aids that give body and texture to the food. They include agar-agar, gelatin, cellulose, pectin, and starch. <u>These additives are mostly food-based, are listed on the label, and are generally safe.</u> Examples of their use include gelatin in yogurt (to maintain consistency), and calcium chloride in canned tomatoes (to maintain texture). Carageenan, a seaweed-based additive used in cottage cheese and toothpaste, has raised questions recently because it may be an intestinal irritant.

- **Processing aids and clarifying agents** help to clear bacteria and debris from foods. Gelatin and albumin help to remove small particles of copper or iron from liquids such as beer and vinegar. Tannin from teas is also used to clarify beverages like beer and wine. <u>Most of these additives are unlisted, but are generally safe.</u>

- **Nutritional supplements** include a long list of both natural and synthetic vitamins and minerals used to enrich foods (to add back what was depleted during processing) or fortify them (to add more nutrients than were originally there or add nutrients that were never in the food). The B vitamins are commonly added back into grain and cereal products. Vitamin A is used in margarine, vitamin D in milk, and vitamin C in fruit drinks. Iodine is added to table salt. Recently, folic acid has been added to many products because research indicates that its deficiency can contribute to birth defects.

ENRICHED AND FORTIFIED FOODS

Enriched: *Replaced nutrients that were lost during processing of that specific food,* such as the loss of several B vitamins (thiamine, riboflavin, and niacin) from the refinement of grains to make flour, which then are added back.

Fortified: *The addition of nutrients to a food that were not originally present,* such as adding vitamin D to milk and iron, which is added to a variety of foods.

- Potassium iodide was added to salt beginning in 1924 to help prevent the epidemic of goiter, a thyroid enlargement from iodine deficiency. This was the first case of fortification of our food supply.
- Vitamin D was added to milk in 1933 to prevent rickets, a common bone deformity problem at that time, caused by vitamin D deficiency, particularly in children.
- Thiamine (vitamin B_1) deficiency causes beri-beri, which causes skin and neurological problems. Most B vitamins are lost in the flour refinement process. In 1940, vitamins B_1, B_2 (riboflavin), and B_3 (niacin), along with iron, were added to flour.
- Vitamin C was first added to foods in the 1950s, specifically to Tang and a variety of fruit juices. Hi-C is a popular sugar drink today that contains added vitamin C.
- Folic acid, another B vitamin, is now (starting in 1998) being added to grain-based foods, such as breads, cereals, and pastas, since folate deficiency has finally been documented to cause birth defects.
- The USDA may begin fortifying candy bars and other snack foods with a variety of nutrients, since many Americans consume these caloric foods in significant amounts, as much as 10 to 30% or more of their daily diet.

Health Note: Most breakfast cereals contain added nutrients, which are often sprayed on the food or added to the dough. Most of these nutrients are water-soluble and may end up in the milk. So, to get these extra nutrients, finish your cereal and drink the milk before you head off to school or work. There are, of course, other healthier ways to obtain a nutritious breakfast.

FOOD ADDITIVES TO AVOID

Avoiding toxins in your diet is an initial step toward enhancing your health and lowering your risk of disease. Let's look at the key additives that may undermine your health. Those with immediate effects may cause headaches or alter your energy level, or they may affect your mental concentration, behavior, or immune response. Those with long-term effects could increase your risk of cancer, cardiovascular disease, and other degenerative conditions.

Make a decision to either cut down on or cut out altogether those food additives that may be hazardous to your health. It may seem difficult to change habits and find substitutes for the foods you enjoy, remind yourself that you will be adding wholesome new flavors and foods to your diet that you may come to like just as much or even more. Avoidance and discrimination are crucial proactive steps in most natural health care programs.

12 Key Additives to Avoid (or Eat Only Occasionally)

1. Hydrogenated fats or "junky" fats are my number one no-no. Minimizing your consumption will reduce the risk of chronic disease. Ironically, clever marketing and lack of thorough research had convinced us for some time that it was healthier to consume these artificial fats—margarine was supposedly better than butter. Although we shouldn't consume large amounts of butter, small amounts are okay, whereas we should avoid margarine and other hydrogenated fats and oils. (Hydrogenation infuses polyunsaturated fats with hydrogen, changing their biochemical structure, and thus "saturating" them.) Hydrogenated fats are artificial—they are not found in nature, and are one of the common unnecessary additives of the food industry. It has now been shown that hydrogenated fats are actually hazardous to your health. They increase the risk of cardiovascular diseases and obesity, and generally stress the liver, which must detoxify them.

Reduce any regular use of foods containing significant amounts of hydrogenated fats. These include margarine, most chips, and many manufactured baked goods, such as crackers, cookies and the like. There are some natural food brands that avoid hydrogenated fats, and these are a better choice.

2. Artificial food colors are coloring agents, may of which have carcinogenic properties; many are allergenic and are also believed to contribute to hyperactivity,

12 KEY ADDITIVES TO AVOID AND THEIR HEALTH RISKS

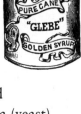

1. **Hydrogenated Fats**—cardiovascular disease, obesity
2. **Artificial Food Colors**—allergies, asthma, hyperactivity; possible carcinogens
3. **Nitrites and Nitrates**—these substances can develop into nitrosamines in the body, which can be carcinogenic
4. **Sulfites** (sulfur dioxide, metabisulfites, and others)— allergic and asthmatic reactions
5. **Sugar and Sweeteners**—obesity, dental cavities, diabetes and hypoglycemia, increased triglycerides (blood fats) or candida (yeast)
6. **Artificial sweeteners** (Aspartame, Acesulfame K, and Saccharin)—behavioral problems, hyperactivity, allergies, and possibly carcinogenic. The government cautions against the use of any artificial sweetener by children and pregnant women. Anyone with PKU (phenylketonuria— problem metabolizing phenylalanine, an amino acid) should not use aspartame (Nutrasweet).
7. **MSG** (monosodium glutamate)—common allergic and behavioral reactions, including headaches, dizziness, chest pains, depression and mood swings; also a possible neurotoxin
8. **Preservatives** (BHA, BHT, EDTA, etc.)—allergic reactions, hyperactivity, possibly cancer-causing; BHT may be toxic to the nervous system and the liver
9. **Artificial Flavors**—allergic or behavioral reactions
10. **Refined Flour**—low-nutrient calories, carbohydrate imbalances, altered insulin production
11. **Salt** (excessive)—fluid retention and blood pressure increases
12. **Olestra** (an artificial fat)—diarrhea and digestive disturbances

Other Concerns

Food Waxes (protective coating of produce, as in cucumbers, peppers, and apples)—may trigger allergies, can contain pesticides, fungicide sprays, or animal byproducts.

Plastic packaging—Carcinogenic (vinyl chloride); immune reactions, lung shock learning problems, and difficulty with concentration in children and in some adults. I strongly recommend avoiding the regular intake of foods that contain artificial colors. This is especially important for our children, who seem to gravitate to the brightly-colored artificial foods that pervade our food industry. Foods to avoid include colored drinks, color-coated candies, gummy and chewy candies, most colored cereals, and cookies and cakes with colorful toppings. Most of these "foods" are also heavily sweetened and not particularly nutritious. **Be extra aware of these additives when shopping at candy counters or vending machines. And be especially mindful of food choices on holidays, such as Christmas, Halloween, and birthdays.**

3. Nitrites and nitrates are preservatives that can be converted to nitrosamines in our body, and research indicates that these compounds can be highly carcinogenic. Vitamin C seems to be protective against this process, so it is suggested that any time you eat nitrated and nitrited foods, take at least 500 to 1,000 mg of vitamin C. (Little packets of vitamin C powder are available that you can carry in your pocket or purse.) Nitrites and nitrates are found most often in preserved meats and lunchmeats such as hot dogs, bologna, bacon, and salami. **Overall, it is wisest to avoid these smoked and preserved meats altogether because they are also sources of saturated fats, meat contaminants, and added chemicals.**

4. Sulfites (such as sulfur dioxide in fruits, sulfites in grapes and wines, and metabisulfites in other foods) are common agents that are now limited to preserving dried fruits and freshly cut potatoes, and in fruit juice concentrates; they are also sprayed on grapes and commonly used in making wine. Sulfites are known to trigger allergic reactions in sensitive individuals. Anyone suffering from allergies or asthma should avoid sulfited foods, while others should keep exposures to a minimum. Sulfites can cause headaches, nausea or diarrhea, irritated membranes, and allergic reactions, particularly in people with asthma. **In people prone to certain forms of asthma, sulfites have, on occasion, triggered anaphylactic shock. The FDA receives hundreds of reports yearly regarding sulfite reactions.**

5. Sugar and natural sweeteners show up in a staggering variety of food products. Common problems from overuse include dental caries, obesity and its associated consequences, diabetes and the secondary effects of elevated blood sugar, hypoglycemia, behavioral changes, such as hyperactivity or difficulty concentrating, yeast problems, excessive food cravings, and more. (You may refer to Chapter 5 on Sugar Detoxification in my book, *The Detox Diet,* for further information on the sugar problem.) Even natural sweeteners should be limited to no more than 10% of your diet. These include honey, maple syrup, date sugar, brown rice syrup, barley malt, fruit juice and fruit juice concentrates, fructose, sucanat (cane sugar juice), and molasses. **Notice the effects on your body and mood during the hours following your consumption of sweeteners. Do your mood and energy levels rapidly improve and then suddenly drop? At that point, do you experience irritability, depression, or both? Or sleepiness or anxiety? Wouldn't you like to avoid the inevitable lows that follow the initial "high" of sugar consumption?**

6. **Artificial sweeteners** such as aspartame, saccharin, and acesulfame K are synthetic sweeteners. **Avoid using them regularly or in large quantities. Saccharin** is the greatest concern, but it is less available these days, so high exposures are not likely. Research studies have linked saccharin with cancer in laboratory animals as both a cancer initiator and promoter. It has also caused fatal genetic mutations in animal studies. **Aspartame** is widely used throughout the diet industry, in soft drinks, chewing gum, candies, and other products. Two research studies found it caused brain tumors in lab animals. It does have some calories and some people may be hypersensitive or show reactions after its use. Aspartame is contraindicated in individuals with PKU, pregnant women, and children under seven. **Acesulfame K** (Ace-K) is a more recently developed sweetener marketed as the brands Sunette and Sweet One. It is 200 times sweeter than sugar and is utilized as a sweetener and as an additive in chewing gum, beverage mixes, instant tea and coffee, non-dairy creamers, and desserts. It has been found to cause brain tumors in animals.

7. **MSG** (monosodium glutamate) is the flavor enhancer linked to the common reactions referred to as "Chinese Restaurant Syndrome," including headaches, agitation, increased heart rate, tightness in the chest, and tingling muscles or skin. Some restaurants avoid using MSG and even advertise that they do so. **Avoid the regular intake of the many products that contain this flavor enhancer, from soups and crackers, to candies and a variety of other processed foods. To avoid this one, you will need to read the labels.**

8. **Preservatives,** such as BHA, BHT, and EDTA, are used only in small quantities in grain products (cereals and crackers), soup bases, and other food products containing oils to prevent rancidity and to preserve freshness. Preservatives are chemicals that must be processed by our body and are potentially toxic to the liver and kidneys. They are known to cause allergic reactions and neurotoxic effects, and in

research studies, BHA and BHT have caused cancer. (BHT is prohibited as a food additive in England.) EDTA doesn't seem to be quite as harmful as BHT and BHA. **Children can be sensitive to preservatives, may demonstrate hyperactivity and behavioral changes, and should avoid regular use. In general, it is best to limit preserved foods since the freshest foods tend to be the most nutritious.**

9. **Artificial flavors** represent the largest number of additives, the majority of which we don't really need. Most of the products that contain artificial flavoring are industrially processed, highly refined, and best limited to an occasional treat. **Adults and children may exhibit a variety of behavioral and allergic reactions to these chemical flavorings.**

10. **Refined flour**, although not officially a food additive, can encourage weight gain and is a main cause of obesity when overused. It is an unnecessary "additive" to our diet. Refined flours (processed grains) are typically used in products such as breads, cereals, cakes, cookies, doughnuts, crackers, and croissants in place of more complete and nutritious whole grain products. The lower fiber content of refined flour can lead to a variety of digestive problems, from constipation to diverticulitis. Eating some refined flour products as an occasional treat is less of a problem within a high-fiber, natural foods diet. **There are many delicious whole grain products now available; these include breads, cereals, pastas, crackers, and cookies, as well as wheat-free corn- and rice-based products. Whatever the source, be sure to check the carbohydrate content on the label to avoid taking in excessive calories and carbohydrates.**

11. **Salt**, or sodium chloride, is needed by our bodies for strength and the proper electrical conductivity within cells. Eating too much salt can lead to fluid retention and increased blood pressure. Emotional irritability also may be associated with high salt intake. Too much salt can also influence a woman's menstrual cycle. **From the perspective of Chinese medicine, excess use or desire for salty foods may represent an imbalance in the body, signifying potential problems in the kidneys and bladder.**

12. **Olestra** is a newly synthesized fat substitute intended to meet the public's desire to stay trim or lose weight, while still eating rich-tasting foods. Olestra is currently being marketed in selected products, including a new potato chip, which has only half the calories (75 versus 150 calories per ounce) of the regular high-calorie, high-

fat chips. If you must eat potato chips, these are an improvement in terms of calories, or you could just eat half the chips you usually eat. Either way, potato chips should only be eaten as a special treat. **Since Olestra is a nonabsorbable oil polymer, it's not really metabolized by the body. Consumer reports indicate that it causes mainly digestive problems, including abdominal cramping, diarrhea, and fecal incontinence. I don't plan on trying this product myself.**

Other Food Additive Problems

Food waxes are usually oil or hydrocarbon based and are not digestible or usable by our bodies. They are used on produce as a protective covering and to hold in moisture, most commonly on cucumbers and apples. Although they are not terribly toxic in and of themselves, they may contain other chemical toxins, such as pesticides, mold inhibitors, and other additives, and **are best avoided.**

Food packaging comes in many forms. Plastic packaging, such as polyvinyl chloride (a potentially carcinogenic chemical) and polyethylene, painted boxes and papers, all introduce additional toxins directly into our food, and many are carcinogenic. In addition, food wraps may out-gas (discharge) plastic toxins into the foods. Many grocery stores seal meats, poultry, fish, and other foods in this plastic wrap using heat, which releases the polyvinyl chloride (PVC) as a gas. **We can limit our exposure to these chemicals by eating fewer packaged and plastic-wrapped foods.**

On the Label or Not?

Let's take a closer look now at how chemicals are used by food manufacturers. During processing, fruits, vegetables, whole grains, and other foods are ground, mashed, boiled, and otherwise manipulated to create the multitude of boxed, canned, packaged, and plastic wrapped "foods" that we find in our stores.

Chemicals are added to foods in a number of ways. First, there are the intentional additives that become ingredients in our foods. These chemicals are the only ones we will see listed on the packages. Sadly however, there are also many additives that never appear on our "truth-in-packaging" labels; these are classified as "indirect additives." The packaging itself can also pose a danger of contamination, since various chemicals and metals are used in their production.

These secondary contaminants (really "hidden" ingredients) such as chemicals used during processing, additives already in pre-prepared ingredients, and chemicals used in packaging, may all wind up in our foods as well. Hidden additives that may be contained in other ingredients include possible toxins in lard or in MSG, both of which are routinely added to already prepared foods, but rarely disclosed on the label.

Finally, there are the "silent additives," which can also be a serious concern: pesticides, pollutants, antibiotics, hormones, and other drugs given to animals or found in animal feed; chemicals in the water and air; and other ever-present industrial chemical pollutants. The best way to prevent harm from these "economic poisons" is to prohibit their use in the first place.

It sometimes seems that there is more concern about chemical exposures in the home or at work than about the chemical danger in eating common food. Replacing dirt and germs with chemicals has been part of twentieth-century living.

Although the chemicals used as food additives are closely regulated by the FDA and seem to pose less short-term risk, we do not really know the risks posed by their long-term use. We are routinely exposed to so many different subtle toxins that when we develop certain health problems, it can be difficult to isolate a specific chemical or other factors that may have been responsible.

Are These Additives Safe?

Just because certain food additives are still in use today and hence have been deemed "safe" doesn't mean that they really are. We need to remember that there is little research on possible long-range effects of food additives, just as we lack information on the cumulative effects of pesticides. One of the FDA's roles is to request and review research data regarding both chemicals currently in use as well as potential new ones. It has the authority to change the status of any chemical used in food, remove old ones from use, or approve new ones. Additives that have been found to be unsafe and which have been removed after years of use include Red Dye #2, cyclamate (artificial sweetener), and cobalt sulfate. From 1949 to 1982, 26 additives and artificial colors were banned from use in foods, following extensive research. But, alarmingly, since 1982, no more bans have been implemented, despite the large number of new chemicals introduced and the list of substances on probationary status, such as aspartame and ace-K (artificial sweeteners) and olestra (an artificial fat).

There are currently about 3,000 food additives approved for use in the foods we eat or the beverages we drink. The average American annually consumes about 150 pounds of sweeteners from sugars and corn sweetener (1995 figures). In 1995, almost 40 billion pounds of sweeteners were consumed in the U.S. In addition, salt intake is about 15 pounds per year per person, while various other food additives account for another 5 to 10 pounds. Sweeteners and other additives have boosted the success of both the "junk food" and "fast food" markets, where the majority of them are consumed.

Food Additives and the Law

In 1958, Congress approved the FDA's "Generally Recognized as Safe" (GRAS) list when it enacted the Delaney Clause, which also required rigid testing for any new food additives and proposed not using any substance that caused cancer in experimental animals. Several thousand additives that were already in use were reviewed by scientists, and those considered safe were placed on the GRAS list. This meant that they were accepted without further testing because there were no specific reports or findings about direct negative effects from these additives. The accepted list included most of those several thousand substances, such as salt, sugar, spices, vitamins, minerals, flavorings, preservatives, emulsifiers, and so on. Some classifications restrict additive levels or their application to certain foods; they are classified as "for intended use based on standard manufacturing processes." Other additives can be used freely.

One of the problems with the GRAS list is lack of knowledge regarding many of the additives that are included. With better testing, some of them have been shown to be unsafe, particularly when increased consumption causes intake to exceed "intended exposure" levels. In 1977, a fairly extensive review of the GRAS list was undertaken; many of the additives are still being investigated. However, their status has not changed, and since 1977, only two additives have been banned—orange B in 1978 (an artificial coloring linked to cancer) and cinnamyl anthranilate in 1982 (an artificial flavoring also linked to cancer).

The safety of these substances on the GRAS list now seems to be taken for granted. According to the FDA, manufacturers are able to use additives on the GRAS list in new applications without an additional specific petition.

During the past ten years, the Delaney Clause has been the subject of media attention and active lobbying to reopen debate on this ruling, which requires the banning for human consumption of any substance causing cancer in lab animals. The food industry points out that accurate comparisons cannot be made between animals and people, and that the large amounts of additives given to animals in a research setting are not directly relevant to the minute amounts of additives used in foods. On the other hand, consumer advocates remind us that the research studies typically last six months, and never more than two years, whereas human cancers may take 20 years to develop. No one really knows the long-term effects of small amounts of chemicals consumed frequently over a lifetime. And the effects on children are an even bigger concern.

Food Additive Health Concerns

In addition to the concern about links between additives and cancer, we cannot yet draw decisive conclusions about the effects of extremely small doses on the brain and nervous system. Some additives, such as MSG, are documented excitotoxins with the capacity to stimulate the brain in unpredictable ways; but we do not know their specific effects, especially on children. Nor is it clear what their actual relationship to hyperactivity or attention deficit disorder (ADD) might be. However, numerous studies and research projects have found that children function and concentrate better when they are on a simpler diet of the right whole foods, avoiding most food additives (Feingold Association).

We also lack information on the role additives play (as mutagens) on our genetic makeup. The food industry questions such concerns and denies that there are any health risks in consuming food additives in small amounts. However, some additives, such as aspartame (the artificial sweetener found in diet sodas and other diet foods), are being consumed, even by young children, in higher than tested amounts.

In addition, there is very little research on the interactive effects of additives because, typically, only one substance is tested at a time. A 1976 study, published in the *Journal of Food Science*, looked at interactive effects. When three additives were tested one at a time, no ill effects were caused in the lab animals (rats). When two of the additives were given together, however, the animals became ill, and when the three were given in combination, all the animals died within 14 days.

What are the real effects on us when we consume, let's say, a ballpark hot dog with sodium nitrite and animal fats, yellow dye #5 in the relish, preservatives in the hot dog bun, and aspartame in the diet soda? I personally don't want to find out, yet many children test this chemical combination daily.

With all the current data and common sense, it's best to follow a "better safe than sorry" approach when it comes to food additives.

The FDA, as our primary governmental watchdog, monitors issues involving food additives. They have thousands of reports on health incidences that have occurred with substances such as MSG and sulfites. Information is frankly provided on their web site (www.fda.gov). For example, in the case of sulfites, which are often a hidden additive, some asthmatics are at risk of life-threatening allergic reactions. At this point, the FDA views its role as one of public education, warning asthmatics to avoid sulfites, rather than further controlling the use of this additive.

Food Irradiation

The Army originally began using irradiated foods in the early 1960s, serving such foods as irradiated bacon, ham, potatoes, and strawberries to personnel on twelve military bases. The FDA later repealed their use after cellular studies suggested that irradiated sugar affected cell growth and produced damaged chromosomes. But food irradiation has come back strong in recent years. As with many low-level radiation studies, it causes no obvious immediate effects on the consumer. Many spices and herbs have been irradiated for years, as has pork, with which there is always a danger of contamination. It is now likely that some grains (irradiated grains have been shipped abroad), fresh fruits and vegetables, and frozen foods are irradiated.

Foods are irradiated, ostensibly, to improve their shelf life and prevent microbial and insect contamination, so that there is less waste and more profits. It can also reduce the use of toxic chemicals to preserve these foods. Irradiation is done by exposing foods to gamma rays emitted from a nuclear source, such as cobalt 60, as they pass on a conveyor belt. It is claimed that the irradiated foods do not themselves become radioactive and thus are not introducing radiation to the consumer.

The concern with food irradiation is that it may produce byproducts that are carcinogenic and increase the incidence of leukemia and other types of cancer or disease of the liver and kidneys. Health problems may not become evident for twenty to thirty years. Most of us are very skeptical about radiation in general, whether it be x-rays or even microwaves, let alone gamma radiation of our food. It is also possible that irradiation may affect the nutritional content of the foods treated, by altering protein structure, reducing vitamin levels, or rendering sensitive enzymes inactive.

FOOD ADDITIVE CHART

SAFE ADDITIVES *(As far as we know)*

Acids—citric, sorbic, lactic

Alginates

Annatto

Beta-carotene or Carotene

Calcium proprionate

Carrageenan

Casein and lactose

Gelatin

Glycerin—mono- and diglycerides

Lecithin

Minerals—iron, zinc, and others

Natural flavoring

Pectin

Potassium sorbate

Sorbitol

Vanillin

Vitamins A, C, and E

ADDITIVES TO LIMIT *(use with caution)*

Aluminum salts

Artificial flavorings

Aspartame

BHA (butylated hydroxyanisole)

Caffeine

EDTA

Gums

Hydrogenated vegetable oils

Polysorbate 60, 65, 80

Propyl gallate

Propylene glycol

Salt

Sodium benzoate

Sugars (sucrose, dextrose, corn syrup)

THBQ

Xylitol

ADDITIVES TO AVOID

Acesulfame K

Artificial colors (FDC colors)

BHT (butylated hydroxytoluene)

BVO (Brominated Vegetable Oil)

MSG (monosodium glutamate)

Olestra

Saccharin

Sodium nitrite and nitrate

Sulfites (especially sodium bisulfite)

Sulfur dioxide

The FDA and the Department of Energy, would like us to believe that food irradiation is a safe process. Actually, they would just like to irradiate foods and not have us know anything about it. There is definite support from the food industry, the nuclear industry, and the U.S. Army to irradiate a wide range of foods. Currently, there is justification for demanding that irradiated food be labeled so the

---

HEALTHY DIET TIPS FOR MINIMIZING ADDITIVES IN YOUR DIET

At least 50% of your diet should be fresh fruit and vegetables.

1. Buy or grow as many of them organically as possible—and start today!
2. Eat more whole grains, beans, nuts, and seeds as the other main components of your diet.
3. Eat seasonally because this will bring your daily life into harmony with the Earth and her cycles and help you to choose the best local produce.
4. Eat primarily locally available foods. This minimizes the chemicals used in shipping, and these foods are usually less costly.
5. Limit your consumption of animal products.
6. Consider manufactured or processed foods, especially fatty and sugary snacks, sodas, and chips, as treats and eat them only occasionally. Notice how you feel when you do eat them.
7. Drink plenty of clean, uncontaminated water.
8. Make a list of what to buy, what to eat, what to grow, and what not to buy or eat. A simple shopping guideline to follow is: "If you can't pronounce it, don't buy it."

---

consumer can choose whether to eat it or not. Do we wish to support a food irradiation industry with the use of recycled nuclear wastes to justify nuclear weapons production?

Is It Necessary to Give Up All Processed Foods and Food Additives?

As I've pointed out in this chapter, some food additives doesn't pose as great a threat as others, and some pose no threat at all. And as far as never, ever eating something that appears on the list of "Additives to Avoid" that follows, here is a sensible rule to start with: If there are special treats that you just can't imagine living without, have them only on occasion. But be aware of what those special treats contain. Think about the possible wholesome alternatives that might taste just as good and which don't put your health at risk. Also, consider changing your consumer habits. Are there farmer's markets in your area where you could shop fre-

---

CENTER FOR SCIENCE IN THE PUBLIC INTEREST

I want to acknowledge the Center for Science in the Public Interest (CSPI), a Washington, DC based consumer advocacy group for safe food that has assessed the research and provides guidelines on food safety. They are clearly on the side of the consumers. You can check their website at *www.cspinet.org* for ongoing updates on nutrition and food additives to avoid. They suggest, "A simple general rule about additives is to avoid sodium nitrite, saccharin, caffeine, olestra, acesulfame K, and artificial coloring. Not only are they among the most questionable additives, but they are used primarily in foods of low nutritional value." And don't forget to minimize sugar and salt.

---

quently? Is there a natural foods market with organic produce nearby that you've never bothered to check out?

Changing your shopping and eating routines isn't something you will do overnight. The first step is to sharpen your awareness about what you're currently eating. Then you can take steps to make the changes you desire for a healthier future.

Take a look at the following charts and decide which food additives and chemicals you want to avoid from now on. All of these substances are discussed more specifically in the Appendix of this book and in Chapter 11 of *Staying Healthy with Nutrition*. **Copy this list and take it with you if you need it as a shopping guide.** Add any of your own concerns to the list, in case you have any allergies, digestive problems, or follow a low-salt, low-sugar, or low-fat diet. Here's to your good health!

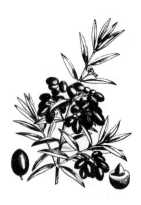

Resources

Books: If you have a deeper interest in this topic, do a little more reading. Ruth Winter has an informative book, *A Consumer's Dictionary of Food Additives* (Three Rivers Press, 1994). It is a thoughtful and thorough review of more than 2,000 additives.

Websites: Check out the information on nutrition on the World Wide Web. The web site most focused on food additives is by the Center for Science in the Public Interest (CSPI) at www.cspinet.org. Your children may enjoy this site as well. It has cooking ideas for kids, cartoon vegetables, and lots of easy-to-understand information. The Center for Science in the Public Interest (CSPI) also produces a very helpful, large and colorful chart, "Chemical Cuisine." They can be contacted at 1501 16th St. NW, Washington, DC 20036.

Organizations: Support the organizations that are your advocates for cleaner food. On the issue of food additives, CSPI and the Feingold Association are excellent resources.

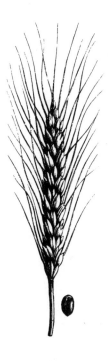

CHAPTER FIVE

Reading Food Labels

◆

Why Is It So Important to Read Food Labels?

Reading a food label takes a little know-how. Given the more than 3,000 additives used in processed foods, it is a challenge to fully understand the risks and benefits of all the ingredients that may appear on a food's label. However, unless you are going to avoid every packaged or processed product, you need to have some basic information on the how-tos of label reading. This chapter will provide you with those basics.

Prior to 1994, food labels provided us only with an ingredients list. The labels we take for granted today have greatly expanded information that can be quite helpful to those with special needs, such as a low-salt diet. Here's a sample food label with the basic components.

As you review the specifics in this chapter, you will come to understand that labels contain important information, such as sugar, fat, and calorie content, that will help you make healthy food choices. Knowing how to read a food label and understanding the benefits and risks of the ingredients listed on it, will

Nutrition Facts

Serving Size 2 crackers (14 g)
Servings Per Container About 21

Amount Per Serving

Calories 60   Calories from Fat 15

	% Daily Value*
Total Fat 1.5g	**2%**
Saturated Fat 0g	**0%**
Polyunsaturated Fat 0g	
Monounsaturated Fat 0.5g	
Cholesterol 0mg	**0%**
Sodium 140mg	**6%**
Total Carbohydrate 10g	**3%**
Dietary Fiber Less than 1g	**3%**
Sugars 0g	
Protein 2g	

Vitamin A 0%	•	Vitamin C 0%
Calcium 0%	•	Iron 2%

* Percent Daily Values are based on a 2,000 calorie diet. Your daily values may be higher or lower depending on your calorie needs:

	Calories:	2,000	2,500
Total Fat	Less than	65g	80g
Sat Fat	Less than	20g	25g
Cholesterol	Less than	300mg	300mg
Sodium	Less than	2400mg	2400mg
Total Carbohydrate		300g	375g
Dietary Fiber		25g	30g

INGREDIENTS: ENRICHED WHEAT FLOUR (CONTAINS NIACIN, REDUCED IRON, THIAMINE MONONITRATE {VITAMIN B1}, RIBOFLAVIN {VITAMIN B2}, FOLIC ACID), CRACKED WHEAT, VEGETABLE SHORTENING (PARTIALLY HYDROGENATED CANOLA AND/OR SOYBEAN OILS), SALT, BAKING SODA, WHEY, MALTED BARLEY FLOUR, YEAST.

enable you to decide if the product is a nutritious and essential food, an occasional treat, or something to be avoided altogether.

Some useful tools for label reading include a magnifying glass, calculator, this book, patience, and perseverance.

THE BASIC FOOD LABEL

Let's look at the key categories of information on a food label and discuss what can be learned from them.

FOOD LABEL CATEGORIES

Serving size

Servings per container

Calories

Calories from fat

Total fat

    Saturated fat

    Polyunsaturated fat

    Monosaturated fat

Cholesterol

Sodium

Total Carbohydrate

    Dietary fiber

    Sugars

Protein

Other nutrients

    Vitamin A

    Vitamin C

    Calcium

    Iron

    Others

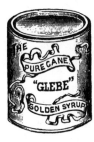

Serving Size *is the calculation upon which all the other numbers on the food label are based.* The food manufacturer often tries to limit the serving size so that the amount of calories or fat will appear smaller, especially in foods such as chips or cookies. For example, they might declare a serving as one or two cookies or an ounce of potato or corn chips when, in reality, the consumer is likely to consume much more at any one time.

So, if you are considering eating "the whole thing," check out the label. You may want to bring your calculator—because you'll need to multiply the serving size by the number of servings in the package to determine the actual amount of calories, fat, and carbohydrate you might consume. Also, see the examples discussed later in this chapter.

Servings Per Container *is the number that lets you know the multiplication factor, should you decide to consume several servings or the entire package.* For example, an 8-ounce bag of potato chips, which lists 150 calories for a 1-ounce serving, actually contains a whopping 1200 calories if you eat the whole bag! And that includes about 500 calories of fat! And then we wonder why it's so easy to be overweight!

Calories *is the figure that represents the number of calories in one serving.* A calorie is a unit of energy or heat that your body generates from the food you eat. The body requires calories to run. It converts carbohydrates, proteins, and fats (the macronutrients from which we get calories) into glucose, the essential fuel for our system. If we take in an excess number of calories, especially sugars and starches, they are stored in the body as fat, and this can lead to weight gain and obesity unless we exercise sufficiently to burn them. Being chronically overweight can be a primary cause of illness and chronic disease.

One of the keys to good nutrition is to consume primarily wholesome foods that are high in nutrients. The objective is to eat mostly foods with a high nutrient-to-calorie ratio, such as certain vegetables that are low in calories and high in vitamins and minerals. Seafood also has many quality nutrients and proteins, without excessive calories or much fat; in fact, the fats in fish are known to be healthful. In contrast, processed and packaged foods are lower in nutrients and often have too many calories and fats. Even the fat-free foods designed for low-fat diets contain higher levels of sugar and carbohydrate and thus more calories—not ideal for long-term health, balanced brains, and trim bodies.

For a better diet plan, consume the majority of your calories from natural and whole foods—fresh fruits and vegetables, whole grains, beans, nuts and seeds, fish and poultry, and low-fat or nonfat dairy products.

Calories from Carbohydrates *are not listed at the top of the label* (you can get this total by multiplying the total grams of carbohydrates by 4 calories). By listing only total calories and fat calories, food manufacturers give us a false sense of security—the sense that if we eat only low-fat products, we are limiting all the foods that might cause excessive weight gain and health problems. But eating too many refined carbohydrates (sweets and starches) can cause weight gain and subsequent degenerative diseases, just as fats do.

Calories from Fat *is listed right after the number of calories, and signifies the total number of fat calories per serving.* This is important information for people who are watching their fat intake and calories. The kind of fat you eat also matters. Much of the fat we consume from processed foods, including saturated and hydrogenated fats, lacks the essential fatty acids our body needs. And typically, eating foods with higher amounts of these unhealthy fats is linked to heart disease and stroke.

Beware of the "junky fats" (mainly hydrogenated and saturated fats) found in fried foods, in baked goods from cookies to crackers to donuts and croissants, in potato or corn chips, and in fatty meats such as salami or bologna. In these high-fat, high-calorie foods, often more than half the calories come from fat. Also, remember that the fats in foods, especially animal-based foods (meat and milk products), store more of the pesticides and chemicals used in their production. So, higher fat foods should be in your "occasional treat" category.

"Calories from Fat" on the label also lets you know the percentage of fat in the product. You'll just have to do some simple math. For instance, in a bag of corn chips that we sampled, there were 150 calories for each 1-ounce serving and 60 calories of fat; that means those chips contained 40% fat. Since the government currently suggests that our diet contain no more than 30% fat (and 20 to 25% is probably more desirable), you may want to avoid foods that have a higher fat content. Obviously, foods such as good quality, cold-pressed vegetable oils or healthy salad dressings are exceptions.

Total Fat *signifies the total grams of fat in each serving of the food.* The label also tells what percent of the day's total ideal fat intake, termed **% Daily Value**, is fulfilled by a single serving of the labeled food. *Government guidelines suggest that our total fat intake be about 60 grams, 540 calories; that is 30% of an estimated 1800-calorie diet.* This may be too high, however realistic, for the optimum health of many people, especially those attempting to restrict fat in their diet.

Saturated Fat *indicates the total grams of saturated fat per serving.* Multiply this figure by 9 to get the saturated fat calories. You definitely want to limit this type of fat, which is primarily found in animal products. It is implicated in atherosclerosis and cardiovascular diseases, and many types of cancer. Hydrogenated fats (found in margarines and many chips and crackers) are also saturated (artificially) and can contribute to these diseases as well.

The % Daily Value allows for 25 grams of saturated fats—this is estimated at about 10-15% of the average food intake.

Polyunsaturated Fat *signifies the total number of grams of polyunsaturated fats per serving.* Polyunsaturates are primarily contained in vegetable oils. Ingredients that come from vegetable shortening or oils other than canola and olive are primarily polyunsaturated fats. Because these fats are less stable biochemically, they tend to oxidize and become rancid more easily than other oils. As a result, foods containing these oils often need preservatives and antioxidants to protect their stability. Such is the case in most salad dressings, crackers, chips and many other baked and packaged goods. *Polyunsaturated fats are not required to be listed on the label; their listing is voluntary.*

NOTE on Hydrogenated Fats: Hydrogenated fats and oils, which should generally be avoided, are not described in this part of the label; they are only listed in the ingredient section. The instability of polyunsaturates is the primary reason the food industry substitutes hydrogenated fats in processed foods—hydrogenation makes fats more stable. Unfortunately, hydrogenated fats can act as irritants, generating free-radicals, which have been implicated in cancer and cardiovascular disease.

Monounsaturated Fats *signifies the number of grams of monounsaturated fats in each serving.* These are healthy fats found in vegetable oils such as olive, canola, or peanut oil. They are more stable, with less of a tendency to become rancid. Their listing is also voluntary, and no % Daily Value is indicated. We should consume more of the healthier monounsaturated fats and fewer saturated and polyunsaturated ones. Women going through menopause can especially benefit from this advice. Monounsaturated fats also support cholesterol balance and don't raise it as saturated fats do.

Cholesterol *indicates the number of milligrams of cholesterol per serving.* This figure reflects the presence of a particular animal fat (sterol) in the product. Food cholesterol is different from body cholesterols. There are both helpful and problematic types of cholesterol in the body, namely HDL (beneficial high-density lipoprotein) and LDL (potentially harmful, low-density lipoprotein). There is clear consensus in medicine and nutrition that it is important to limit the amount of cholesterol we eat. Saturated and hydrogenated fats seem to increase harmful blood cholesterol levels, whereas more healthful monounsaturated fats and fish oils may increase positive cholesterol (HDLs) in the body.

GENERAL NUTRIENT GUIDELINES

Component	Daily Value	Ideal Total Daily Intake	Daily Intake in Calories	Percent of 1800-Cal Diet
Protein	60 grams	50-75 grams	250-300	15-20%
Carbohydrates	300 grams	200-300 grams	800-1,200	50-70%
Fat	60 grams	40-60 grams	350-540	30%
Saturated Fat	25 grams	0-25 grams	0-225	0-15%
Polyunsaturated Fat	Voluntary listing	10-25 grams	100-200	5-10%
Monounsaturated Fat	Voluntary listing	10-25 grams	100-200	5-10%
Cholesterol	300 mg	0-300 mg	minimal	minimal

Sodium *represents the amount of sodium in each serving.* (Sodium is one of the minerals in salt, which is sodium chloride.) Many processed foods, such as crackers, canned soups, packaged meats, and potato or other chips have fairly high amounts of sodium. The Total Daily Value acceptable for sodium is 2,500 mg; this amount can be quite easy to surpass, especially if you have a taste for salty foods or add salt to your meals. Restaurant foods and fast foods are often high in this most common flavor enhancer. People on low-sodium diets will want to watch this category carefully, especially those with high blood pressure, heart disease, or problems with fluid retention.

NOTE: On a food package, "reduced sodium" indicates 25% less sodium content then the "normal" version of that food; "light in sodium" means the sodium has been reduced by at least 50%; "low-sodium" means the food has 140 mg or less per serving; "very low sodium," 35 mg or less; and "sodium-free" means the food has less than 5 mg per serving.

Total Carbohydrates *signifies the number of grams of carbohydrate in each serving.* Carbohydrates include starches, sugars, and dietary fiber. These contribute 4 calories of energy per gram. Carbohydrates include simple sugars such as glucose, fructose (the natural sugar found in fruits), complex starches in whole wheat and brown rice, and dietary fiber. The Total Daily Value for carbohydrate appears to about 300 grams (about 1200 calories and nearly 60% of the average diet), and the label may list the percentage of that amount.

Read the serving size carefully to be sure of how much carbohydrate you are getting in what you eat. For example, a loaf of whole grain bread listed a serving size as one piece, but most people typically will eat at least two slices as a single serving. Knowing your total carbohydrate content means multiplying the number of servings consumed by the number of carbs per serving.

Eating too many carbohydrates (fruits, juices, sweets, and starches) in the diet is one of the greatest risk factors for obesity, and can cause rapid mood swings. Refined carbohydrates are less healthy than complex carbohydrates (whole grains and their products). Processed, refined carbohydrates include products made with refined flour and sugar, such as white breads, white rice, and most pastas; a majority of baked goods are also refined, including cookies, cakes, donuts, crackers; as well as foods high in sweeteners, like sodas, candy, and ice cream. Too many of these sweets or simple sugars can overtax the body's insulin activity. **A diet high in refined carbohydrates has been associated with hypoglycemia problems, diabetes, or atherosclerosis, and subsequent cardiovascular problems.**

Eating more wholesome complex carbohydrate foods—whole grains, such as brown rice, oats, and whole wheat, whole grain pastas, and root vegetables—results in better carbohydrate utilization by the body and more nutrients per calorie.

Dietary Fiber *indicates the number of grams of fiber per serving.* Since fiber is important for preventing diseases and supporting proper colon health, it is specifically listed. However, this entry applies primarily to fiber added back into processed foods, which typically contain only small amounts of fiber compared to whole foods. Fresh fruits and vegetables, whole grains, and beans are high in natural fiber, and are a healthier alternative to packaged processed foods. The minimal suggested daily intake for dietary fiber is 25 to 30 grams.

Sugars *refers to the number of grams of simple sugar in each serving of the product.* Multiplying by 4 calories per gram provides the total calories from sugars. Sugar content refers not only to sweeteners added to the product, but also to sugars that occur naturally, such as fructose in fruits and lactose in milk. This is one of the key areas to monitor in order to maintain good health. Limiting refined sugar intake and lowering all simple sugars is very important. Also, remember to limit even sugars from juices and natural sweeteners, while increasing your complex carbohydrate intake. Try to moderate your intake of both manmade sweeteners—cane and beet sugars (refined), corn syrup, corn sweeteners, fructose, and the artificial aspartame and saccharin—as well as natural sugars—honey, maple syrup, malt, molasses, rice syrup, fruit juice concentrates, and dried fruits. *The majority of the simple sugars in our diet should come from fresh fruits.*

Protein *indicates the number of grams of protein in each serving.* Protein is an essential nutrient that comes primarily from animal tissues, legumes (beans and tofu), nuts and seeds, and dairy products. We can also obtain complete proteins by combining plants, such as rice or corn with beans. (Complete protein means we're getting all the essential amino acids, the building blocks of protein.) Almost all foods, even fruits and vegetables, actually contain some amino acids. We require a certain amount of protein, based on our individual body needs, activity level, and state of health.

Protein deficiency can cause problems, such as fatigue, hypoglycemia, and less resistance to disease. Excess protein, on the other hand, can create problems of long-term toxicity from overconsumption of these more concentrated foods. They make the body overly acidic, which may promote osteoporosis and other metabolic imbalances. We need at least 40 to 50 grams of dietary protein a day, or roughly 1 ounce of protein for every 50 pounds of body weight. One needs additional protein during pregnancy, pre- and post-surgery, when engaging in lots of exercise or body-building, or when recovering from illness.

Other Nutrients *indicates some of the essential vitamins and minerals.* Most food labels include four items: vitamin A, vitamin C, calcium, and iron. It is important to remember that individual requirements for nutrients are unique to each body, and that optimum levels of intake are often higher than government standards for the minimal requirements to prevent deficiency. Like protein and all nutrients, our requirements for vitamins A and C increase when we are ill or under other special circumstances. Our needs for calcium and iron are also unique depending on gender (women usually need more) and on our stage in life. Therefore, if these values are going to be useful, we need to understand these issues more completely.

Vitamin A is an important nutrient for healthy tissue and skin, for immune function, and to help fight infections. Both vitamin A and beta-carotene, a precursor of vitamin A, are included in this category; these two nutrients tend to be interactive. The basic requirement for vitamin A is 5,000 IUs, and there is no specific requirement for beta-carotene even though it is an important antioxidant nutrient found in fresh fruits and vegetables. There seems to be a growing consensus that a variety of carotenes or mixed carotenoids may be the most beneficial.

Vitamin C is one of the most important nutrients for staying healthy. This water-soluble vitamin is an essential antioxidant protecting against many toxins. It also helps our body fight disease and is used in nutritional medicine for a variety of therapies. Government guidelines suggest a minimum daily requirement of 60 mg; my experience indicates, however, that many people do best with 1,000 to 3,000 mg daily, which means that they need to take vitamin C supplements. Nutritional supplementation, especially with a useful antioxidant like vitamin C, helps to buffer against harmful free radicals generated from chemical exposure. Your doctor can advise you concerning your own requirements.

Calcium is an important nutrient that helps strengthen bones and support functions relating to cell metabolism and electrical conductivity. The daily requirement for calcium is 850 mg, but this may vary depending on gender, menopausal status, and other factors.

Iron is needed for making hemoglobin, which carries oxygen in our red blood cells. Men and women have different requirements; men need about 10 mg a day, while menstruating women need 18 mg. Pregnant women need more; postmenopausal women require less. All requirements depend on the blood count and iron status in the body.

Other nutrients that may be listed on a food label include Vitamins D and E, Niacin (vitamin B_3), Phosphorus, or Zinc.

List of Ingredients on the Label

The food's contents are listed in order by quantity—the largest ingredient in the product is listed first, the smallest last. This is an important point. Recently, my family found an "all-organic" treat which sounded healthy, but it contained more sugar than anything else. Sugar was the very first ingredient listed on the label. The ingredient list is also where the "direct additives" are listed—the additives allowed by the FDA as part of the product. See Appendix for specific information.

Using the Label to Avoid Disease

Thousands of research studies have found that there is a very real link between what we eat and our health. Various reports suggest that at least one third to one half of all cases of cancer and heart disease in the United States are directly contributed to by diets high in fat and chemicals and low in fiber. Food labels provide information that can help us choose our food wisely, and thereby reduce the risk of heart disease and cancer and help cope with specific health conditions. Let's look at a few common health concerns and how they are affected by various dietary factors.

Allergies

As we have discussed, not all additives are safe for everyone, so be sure to read the ingredients carefully if you or a family member suffer from allergies, reactive digestive problems, or lactose intolerance. People with asthma could experience strong reactions to sulfites, as serious as anaphylactic shock. Others react adversely to MSG, experiencing a sense of faintness or chest pains. And many people are allergic to citrus fruits, dairy products, eggs, or wheat. Clear labeling information helps you to avoid any allergens you know about.

High Blood Pressure

Nearly 50 million Americans suffer from high blood pressure (hypertension), and many others are at risk. Food labels can be especially helpful with this concern, since the label states the amount of salt (sodium) per serving. Keeping sodium at reasonable intake levels is one important key to controlling high blood pressure. Sodium in a number of forms is often added during food processing, and it is also present naturally in foods such as milk, cheese, meat, fish, and certain vegetables. High blood pressure is more common in overweight people, those with high cholesterol, and those who consume excessive fats in their diet. Anyone with a tendency to hypertension should watch calorie and fat intake as well as their sodium level. The food label can also be used to monitor fat, calories, and carbohydrate intake to limit weight gain, important because obesity is a causative factor in hypertension.

UNDERSTANDING FOOD LABEL TERMS

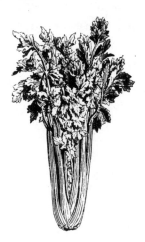

- **Fats**

Fat-free: less than 0.5 g of fat per serving

Low-fat: 3 g of fat or less per serving

Reduced-fat: at least 25% less fat than the correlating food

- **Cholesterol**

Cholesterol-free: less than 2 mg of cholesterol and 2 g or
less of saturated fat per serving

Low-cholesterol: 20 mg or less of cholesterol and 2 g or
less of saturated fat per serving

Reduced or less cholesterol: at least 25% less cholesterol
than the reference (similar) food and 2 g or less of
saturated fat per serving

- **Meats**

Lean: less than 10 g of fat, 4.5 g of saturated fat, and less than 95 mg of cholesterol
per serving

Extra lean: less than 5 g of total fat, less than 2 g of saturated fat, and less than 95
mg of cholesterol per 100 grams

- **Healthy**

Low-fat and Light (two meanings, (1) pertaining to fat, (2) to fat and sodium):

   (1) one-third fewer calories or half the fat of the reference food. If the food
derives 50% or more of its calories from fat, the reduction must be at least
50% of the fat.

   (2) a low-calorie or low-fat food whose sodium has been reduced by at least
50% of the reference food. "Light in sodium" is used when the food has 50%
or less sodium than the reference food but does not meet the restrictions for
calories and fat.

- **Calories**

Calorie-free: fewer than 5 calories per serving

Low-calorie: 40 or fewer calories per serving

Reduced or fewer calories: at least 25% fewer calories than the reference food

- **Fiber**

High-fiber: 5 g or more of fiber per serving

Good source of fiber: 2.5 to 4.9 g of fiber per serving

More or added fiber: at least 2.5 g more fiber per serving than the reference food

* Foods making claims about increased fiber content also must meet the requirements for "low-fat," or the amount of fat per serving must appear next to the claim.

- **Sugar**

Sugar-free: less than 0.5 g of sugar per serving

No added sugar, without added sugar, or no sugar added: no sugar or sugar substitutes (for example, corn syrup or fruit juice) added during processing or packing; or no ingredients made with added sugars, such as jams, jellies, or concentrated fruit juice.

- **Sodium or Salt**

Sodium-free or Salt-free: less than 5 mg of sodium or salt per serving

Very low sodium or salt: 35 mg or less of sodium or salt per serving

Low-sodium: 140 mg of sodium or less per serving

Light in sodium: at least 50% or less sodium per serving than the average reference amount for the same food with no sodium reduction.

Lightly salted: at least 50% less sodium per serving than the reference food

Reduced or less sodium: at least 25% less per serving than the reference food

- **Potassium**

High-potassium: 700 mg or more of potassium per serving

Good source of potassium: 350 to 665 mg of potassium per serving

More or added potassium: at least 350 mg more potassium per serving than the reference food

- **Calcium**

High-calcium: 200 mg or more of calcium per serving

Good source of calcium: 100 to 190 mg of calcium per serving

More or added calcium: at least 100 mg more calcium per serving than the reference food

Heart Disease

If the label makes a claim about the relationship of diet to heart disease, the food must be low in total fats, saturated fat, and cholesterol, since high intake in any of these categories is linked to elevated blood cholesterol and increased risk of coronary artery disease, our most common degenerative disease. *The current general recommendation is to limit fats to 30% or less of the day's nutritional intake, with saturated fat limited to 10% of total calories. (For a 2,000 calorie diet, that amounts to about 65 grams of fat per day and only 20 grams of saturated fat.)* People with extremely high blood cholesterol or with existing heart disease may need to limit fat intake still further, based on their doctor's recommendation. For example, the diet recommended by Dr. Dean Ornish for reversing and preventing heart disease allows only 10% fat, all from unsaturated sources. You would also want to monitor other nutrients, such as sodium and fiber, to support a low-salt, high-fiber diet.

Diabetes

Labeling information can also be vital to people with diabetes, because diet is very important in controlling this condition. Poorly managed diabetes can greatly increase the risk of cardiovascular disease, so diabetics need to monitor fat intake, especially saturated fat and cholesterol. In addition, of course, diabetics should limit their intake of sweets and refined starches in order to stabilize their blood sugar.

LABEL EXAMPLES

The following are examples of the kind of information found on the labels of some common foods. I have noted the categories, grams, percentages, and ingredients that are listed and then analyzed the information in terms of what it reveals about the food's health risks or benefits. I have chosen a selection of common products you might find in your shopping cart, cupboard, or tummy. Look through your pantry or refrigerator, and try your own analysis.

Note: Food items are rated for easy reference.

> ★ — Avoid
> ★★ — Eat occasionally
> ★★★ — Fairly good food
> ★★★★ — Good for regular consumption

Tuna (canned name-brand, packed in water) ★★

Ingredients: Solid white tuna, spring water, hydrolyzed casein, hydrolyzed soy protein, vegetable broth, salt, pyrophosphate.

Comments: This can of tuna actually contains more than the label suggests. The tuna is not just "packed in spring water." There is also added salt and milk- and soy-based hydrolysates, so anyone allergic to milk (the casein molecule) or soy may react to this tuna fish. The pyrophosphate, which sounds more explosive than it actually is, is relatively benign. Additionally, whatever hidden ingredients in the ocean, such as mercury, that might have been absorbed into the tuna may also be in your meal. (Tuna packed in oil has a higher fat and calorie count.)

The can is 6 ounces, and a serving size is 2 ounces, yet the can provides 2.5 servings, so an ounce must be lost in the liquids. Therefore, there are actually 5 ounces of tuna. Tuna is a low-calorie, high-protein food. There are 70 calories per serving, so the whole can only has about 175 calories. There are 10 fat calories; only 1 fat gram, and no saturated fat. Cholesterol is 25 mg and sodium is 250 mg—neither very high. There are 15 grams of protein per serving—that's 60 calories—and no carbohydrates. So this food is made up of mostly protein calories. In fact the whole can of tuna, which is not that difficult to consume, is about 40 grams of protein, nearly the amount of protein that most of us need in a day. Served with a nice green salad and sliced veggies, tuna offers a high-nutrient meal.

Salad Dressing ★★

This is a typical dressing—honey-mustard—found in the health section of the market. Most all basic salad dressings are high in fat.

Ingredients: Canadian canola oil, water, dijon mustard, honey, sugar, white vinegar, onions, apple cider vinegar, salt, turmeric (a natural color), sodium benzoate to preserve freshness, xanthan gum, citric acid.

Comments: This salad dressing actually has better quality ingredients than most. Sodium benzoate (a preservative) and xanthan gum (a thickener) are considered safer than other alternatives. The canola oil is also primarily a monounsaturated fat, a healthier choice than other oils. However, this dressing is still very caloric and over 80% fat, and it contains two sweeteners—honey and sugar.

Serving size is 2 tablespoons, but with the yummy honey and sugar added, you might be tempted to add a little more to your salad. There are 130 calories per serving (or 65 per tablespoon) and 110 calories from fat per serving. The Total Fat is 12 grams per serving; 1 gram from saturated fat, but zero cholesterol because it contains no animal fats. Sodium is 110 mg, lower than many dressings, and Total Carbohydrates are six grams, all from sugars—the added honey and sugar. This is a fairly balanced dressing recipe, but if you find yourself using 4 tablespoons, the fats shoot up to 24 grams, almost half of your daily allotment, and the sugars then add up to 12 grams. There is no protein, and no significant source of fiber or vitamins A and C, calcium, or iron.

Vanilla Soy Milk ★★★

VitaSoy's Vanilla Delite is a nutritious substitute for cow's milk that has become extremely popular in the health food industry. I have chosen the soy milk that my kids like best.

Ingredients: Filtered water, organic whole soybeans, brown rice syrup, barley flour, expeller expressed canola oil, natural vanilla flavor, sea salt.

Comments: This drink contains 190 calories for 8 ounces, and just over 25% fat at 50 fat calories per serving. The 6 grams of fat even have 1 gram of saturated fat from certain fatty acids in the soybeans. However, there is no cholesterol because there are no animal sources. (There are also low-fat soy milks that have removed some of these fats, and lower calorie soy milks than this one without as much sweetener.) This drink has 27 grams of carbohydrates, which represent over 100 calories and 50% of the drink. Most of the carbohydrates are from simple sugars. Also, there are 7 grams of protein, which is pretty good, along with some sodium at 130 mg. This soymilk has about 70 mg of calcium and 1 mg of iron; there are also calcium-enriched soy milks, which are closer in calcium content to cow's milk.

Chocolate, Cream-filled Cookies ★

Ingredients: Sugar, enriched wheat flour (contains niacin, reduced iron, thiamine monohydrate [vitamin B_1], riboflavin [B_2], folic acid), vegetable shortening (partially hydrogenated soybean oil), cocoa, high fructose corn syrup, corn flour, whey, cornstarch, baking soda, salt, soy lecithin (emulsifier), vanillin (an artificial flavor), chocolate.

Comments: Like many cookies, these are mostly sugar and fat, with sugar as the number-one ingredient. To their benefit, they have no artificial food colorings, and they are enriched and fortified with iron and some B vitamins—niacin, thiamine, riboflavin, and folic acid. However, the fats are mostly hydrogenated vegetable oil and some whey (extracted from milk), which are not desirable. And there are 7 grams of fat in each serving of 3 cookies, which provides 160 calories, over 50 calories per cookie. Each serving is comprised of 23 grams of carbohydrate that includes 13 grams of sugar but only 1 gram of dietary fiber, along with 220 mg of sodium. Although there are clearly many higher-fat desserts, the 60 calories of fat per serving along with all the sugar makes the regular consumption of these cookies risky for obesity and cardiovascular problems.

Cereal (Brightly-colored, Sugary Brands) ★

Ingredients: Corn, wheat, and oat flour; sugar, partially hydrogenated vegetable oil (one or more of: coconut, cottonseed, and soybean); salt, sodium ascorbate and ascorbic acid (vitamin C); yellow #6, niacinamide, zinc oxide, reduced iron; natural orange, lemon, cherry, blueberry, raspberry, lime, and other natural flavors; red #40, turmeric color; annatto color; blue #2; pyridoxine hydrochloride (vitamin B_6); blue #1; riboflavin (vitamin B_2); vitamin A palmitate; thiamine hydrochloride (vitamin B_1); BHT (preservative); folic acid (folate); vitamin B_{12} and vitamin D.

Comments: This is a long list, some of which is food, plus a variety of additives and lots of natural flavors and artificial food colors. The cereal companies add some vitamins and minerals, including six B vitamins, some vitamins A, D, and C, plus zinc and iron—11 nutrients in all. Still, a cup of loops provides 120 calories plus whatever the milk adds, and only 10 calories of fat. This is mostly sugar and coloring added to grain flours. The biggest concern I have from this type of cereal is the amount of artificial food colorings. A piece of fresh fruit, such as an apple or banana, would be an excellent addition to this type of cereal for breakfast. Also, many of the added nutrients are sprayed on, so may end up in the milk.

Tomato-based Pasta Sauce ★★★

Ingredients: Tomato purée (water, tomato paste), diced tomatoes, mushrooms, corn syrup, onions, corn oil, salt, roasted garlic (garlic, high maltose corn syrup), parsley, spices, natural flavors.

Comments: One half cup of this sauce provides 110 calories, 12 grams (48 calories) of sugar, and 30 calories of fat, plus 2 grams of protein. It contains small amounts of vitamins C and A, calcium, and iron. Overall, compared to many jarred food products, pasta sauces are fairly nutritious. Let's compare this sauce to an organic, fat-free pasta sauce.

Organic Mushroom Pasta Sauce ★★★★

Ingredients: Organic* tomato puree (tomato paste, filtered water) diced tomatoes, diced onions, raw sugar, mushrooms, garlic, basil, marjoram, parsley, sea salt, black pepper, savory, oregano, thyme, rosemary, bay leaf

Comments: A half cup of this sauce provides 50 calories as 11 grams of carbohydrate, 2 grams of protein, and no fat. This is less than half the calories of the other sauce, the same protein, and no fat. It also has nearly twice the nutrient levels of vitamins A and C, calcium and iron, as well as some other nutrients. Furthermore, we can be pretty certain there are no hidden chemicals in the organic sauce, and it was similarly priced for the same size jar. Although the organic sauce has many health advantages over the conventional sauce, there are many other comparable products with greater differences.

Frozen Lasagna with Meat and Sauce ★

Ingredients: Cooked macaroni (semolina, water), water, tomatoes, low-moisture part-skim mozzarella cheese (part-skim milk, cheese cultures, salt, enzymes), beef, dry curd cottage cheese (cultured skim milk, enzymes), modified cornstarch, salt, parmesan cheese (part-skim milk, cheese cultures, salt, enzymes), bleached enriched wheat flour (wheat flour, niacin, iron, thiamine mononitrate, riboflavin, folic acid), dehydrated onions, sugar, spices, beef flavor (salt, tapioca dextrin, vegetable oil, beef flavor [contains beef extract, smoke flavor], gum arabic, modified cornstarch, citric acid and flavor), dehydrated soy sauce (soybeans, salt, wheat), erythorbic acid, dehydrated garlic, canola oil, natural flavorings, cultured whey, beef stock, caramel coloring.

Comments: Frozen lasagna is made from mostly real food and doesn't have a lot of additives. However, it does have animal fats, is relatively high in fat, and would be even fattier except that it's made with lower fat cheeses. (A non-meat lasagna might have reduced fats and there are several low-fat varieties available in the frozen food section.) Not listed on the label are whatever hidden chemicals that may be present in the meats and dairy products. The small-size package is about 10 ounces and contains 370 calories and 7 grams of saturated fat and 45 mg of cholesterol. It also con-

* Every ingredient has "organic" listed before it.

tains 23 grams of protein, and a variety of vitamins and minerals. It has just over a gram of sodium, 1050 mg per serving. Accompanied by a large green salad (very light on the dressing) or some steamed vegetables, it could be a nourishing meal.

Frozen Vegetables (broccoli, cauliflower and carrots) *in Cheese Sauce* ★

Ingredients: Broccoli, water, cauliflower, carrots, cheeses (cheddar, granular, semisoft and blue cheeses) made from pasteurized milk, cheese cultures, salt, enzymes, annatto (color), contains less than 2% soybean oil, food starch-modified nonfat dry milk, salt, whey, sugar, sodium phosphates, natural flavors, butter (cream, salt), sweet cream buttermilk, xanthan gum, autolyzed yeast extract (may contain MSG), parmesan cheese flavor (milk, cream, water, autolyzed yeast extract, cultures, salt, enzymes), monoglycerides, onion powder, garlic powder, citric acid, yellow 5, yellow 6.

Comments: This long list of ingredients to flavor a half-cup of already cooked vegetables brings its 70-calorie serving to 50% fat. It does have vitamins A and C, and some protein (3 g) from the cheese sauce, and calcium from the broccoli and dairy. We don't need our vegetables to be half fats, including some saturates, cholesterol, and about 500 mg of sodium. The yellow food dyes are not great either and really not necessary. But because this type of dish is more readily accepted by children, it is a viable choice if we can't get our the kids to eat a few veggies any other way.

Fruit Punch Drinks ★

Ingredients: Water, sweeteners (high fructose corn syrup, sugar), apple and grape juices from concentrate, less than 0.5% of natural and artificial flavors, citric acid (provides tartness), ascorbic acid (vitamin C), blue #1 and other dyes.

Comments: This is the new color in the line of juice-flavored (10% fruit juice) sugar water, containing 100 calories of simple sugars in the 7-ounce carton. And it gives a whopping 30 mg of vitamin C. Even though blue artificial colors are not the worst of the synthetic dyes, these drinks are near the bottom of my list of healthful beverage choices.

*NOTE on Chapter 5: For a more in-depth discussion of the food and nutrient categories in this chapter, such as calories, fats and cholesterol, proteins, sugars, dietary fiber, or nutrients like sodium, calcium and iron, refer to Part I of my book, Staying Healthy with Nutrition, *as well as Chapter 15 for nutritional guidelines for you and your family.*

CHAPTER SIX

Walking the Aisles

◆

A TRIP THROUGH THE GROCERY STORE

Many supermarkets offer healthier alternatives to processed, "polluted," and non-nutritious food. Chemical-free and more natural foods are displayed next to processed items, organic choices beside chemically treated and grown produce, and even organic canned and boxed products side-by-side with conventionally packaged foods. I believe that it is vital for each of us to take the time to notice the differences that already exist—in ingredients, chemical additives, nutrient levels, and cost.

In California, for example, major supermarket chains are now offering natural foods and organic produce, and many also provide some organic nuts and grains in bulk. There is one large independent store in my area that features both conventional products, such as cereals, across the same aisle from the natural foods cereals that are made with whole grains, some even organic, without refined sugars, preservatives, and artificial food colors. Certain food manufacturers have responded to this trend as well; for example, two popular brands of baby foods now offer entire lines of organic fruits and vegetables. The trend indicates that these changes are likely to expand in the future as the organic and natural food industries continue to grow.

Let's take an imaginary walk through today's average supermarket and see how you can maximize your food choices. We'll look at typical items on your shopping list—from canned soups to packaged cookies to pasta sauces—and point out nutritional value, ingredients to be cautious of, healthier choices, and in some cases, best options and nutritious additions (what you might do to that particular food to make it healthier).

My goal is to give you realistic options so that buying healthier food for yourself and your family will become an automatic part of your shopping routine. Many of my friends and colleagues have suggested that I advise readers to just stay out of supermarkets altogether so as not to be tempted by all of the commercial, chemicalized foods, and instead to shop exclusively in your garden, at farmer's markets, and at natural food stores (which incidentally also sell a variety of unwholesome, high-calorie high-fat foods, but usually with fewer chemical additives). A more realistic approach is: **shop the perimeter of the supermarket**—the produce section, the meat counters, and the dairy cases, while avoiding the aisles. However, this is not the whole answer either. You'll still have to minimize the higher fat foods and the more heavily treated animal products, even though a popular diet these days focuses on proteins and vegetables. Somewhere, somehow, we need to discover the appropriate balance between shopping and eating healthfully.

Before we take that imaginary walk, review your refrigerator and cupboards before you go shopping so that you can clarify what you need, assess what you have that should be used up, and think of other foods to complement what you already have. Make a shopping list to minimize impulse buying and help you stay within your budget. However, I do encourage trying new foods and recipes and incorporating more fresh foods into your diet.

NOTE: For some fresh and wholesome, made-from-scratch, and easy-to-prepare recipes, refer to my cookbook, *A Diet For All Seasons,* and other healthful cookbooks.

BASIC FOOD CATEGORIES IN THE GROCERY STORE

Note: Food items are rated for easy reference.

★ — Avoid
★★ — Eat only occasionally
★★★ — Fairly good food
★★★★ — Fine for regular consumption

Canned Soups ★★

Nutritional Value: This may vary depending on the type of soup. With grains and veggies, there will be some B vitamins and minerals and dietary fiber; with animal foods, protein; and with cream soups, calcium. Much of the water soluble vitamins, the Bs and C, have been lost from cooking and with storage in the soup cans.

Cautions: MSG, high salt, sugars, and allergens such as wheat and dairy extracts, including casein or sodium caseinate. Cream soups may be high in fats and calories. Some soups may contain chicken and beef remnants (often not the freshest parts) or lard. Note: small cans may actually be 2 servings, so be sure to multiply the calories and fats on the label, depending on how much you consume.

Healthier Choices: Vegetable-based soups that contain all natural products, no MSG, and a minimum of additives.

Nutritious Additions: Add some lightly-cooked fresh veggies and spring water to your can of soup. Or make your own broth by cooking up some vegetables, such as onion, carrots, and potatoes, and add the canned soup to your vegetables. These additions will enhance the flavor and make the soup more nutritious and filling without adding many calories or fats.

Best Options: Organic soups with vegetables.

Canned Chili ★★

Nutritional Value: There is protein in the meat and beans, fiber in the beans and vegetables, and some vitamins and minerals from included veggies and tomato sauce.

Cautions: Lard, poor-quality beef and the chemicals they may include, sugar or corn sweeteners; some may also contain preservatives and MSG.

Healthier Choices: Vegetarian chilis with soy protein, without preservatives; low-fat and lard-free chilis.

Nutritious Additions: Add vegetables, such as onion, bell pepper, carrot, or zucchini with additional water to enhance the chili. Lightly sauté them first and then mix into the chili and heat.

Best Options: Organic vegetarian chili.

Salsas ★★★★

Nutritional Value: Salsas, especially fresh ones, are quite nourishing, although some people find spicy foods irritating. Chilies, tomatoes, cilantro, and onions contain a variety of nutrients. Vitamin C is probably only available in raw (uncooked) salsas.

Cautions: Additives such as sodium benzoate or modified food starch.

Healthier Choices: Freshly made salsas, sometimes available with organic ingredients.

Nutritious Additions: Mix some salsa with salad or with refried beans and make a burrito.

Canned Refried Beans ★★★★

Nutritional Value: These products provide good low-fat protein and dietary fiber. They can be used alone or with rice to make burritos and healthy nachos.
Cautions: May contain lard, an extract of saturated animal fat, or added sugars.
Healthier Choices: Canned vegetarian refried pinto or black beans, either nonfat or with a small amount of canola oil.
Best Options: Canned organic beans, mainly available at the health food store.

Canned Fruits and Vegetables ★★★

Nutritional Value: Heat-stable vitamins and minerals in the fruit or vegetable may stay in the canned produce; however, vitamin C, some B vitamins, and enzymes in the produce will probably be diminished in preparation and lost over time in the can.
Cautions: Added sugars and salts, sugary syrups in fruits, and loss of nutrients in the can.
Healthier Choices: Frozen fruits and vegetables.
Best Options: Fresh fruits and veggies, organic when possible.

Other Canned Foods ★★

Nutritional Value: Some fiber and nutrients are often cooked out or lost in canning.
Cautions: Beware of processed canned foods, meat byproducts, and the many preservatives and additives used in their preparation and packaging.
Healthier Choices: Minimize the use of highly processed canned foods. Dried whole foods that can be soaked, or frozen foods, usually have higher nutrient levels.

Canned and Bottled Tomato Sauces ★★★★

Nutritional Value: A source of beta-carotene, possibly some vitamin C, and other vitamins and minerals contained in tomatoes and other vegetables. These are basically pretty good for regular use.
Cautions: Added sugar and salt, some preservatives.
Healthier Choices: Preservative-free, sugar-free, and organic sauces are ideal, especially with some added veggies in the sauce, such as mushrooms, carrots, zucchini, onion, garlic, and basil.
Best Options: Homemade tomato sauces are ideal. Start with fresh or canned, whole,

or crushed tomatoes. Adding very small pieces of carrots, onion, broccoli, and zucchini to your sauce is a good way to get your kids used to eating a few vegetables.

Ketchup/Catsup ★★

Nutritional Value: Not too much, maybe a few nutrients from the original tomatoes, which are cooked and puréed.
Cautions: This popular American condiment is high in sugar, corn sweeteners, and salt, and should be used in small amounts.
Healthier Choices: Natural ketchups without added sugars, organic ketchups, or good salsas if you like it spicy.
Best Options: For a dish you may normally season with ketchup, try some chopped fresh veggies, such as tomatoes, onion, and bell peppers.

Packaged Whole Grains and Beans ★★★★

Nutritional Value: These are some of your better choices for a whole foods diet. Grains and beans contain a wide variety of vitamins and minerals, as well as amino acids and even some required oils (essential fatty acids) in the germ of the grain. Beans, or legumes, are one of the vegetable proteins, and contain a good amount of dietary fiber. They all need to be cooked in water or sprouted (soaking in water and rinsed once or twice daily to make edible baby plants—very live and nutritious food) to make them edible.
Cautions: The only concern is chemicals that may be used during the growing process, and some companies may spray them (fumigate) before they are packaged to protect them from pests, molds, or premature sprouting. If you are concerned about potential chemical contamination, organic alternatives are available.
Healthier Choices: There aren't many better choices in the grocery store. Organically-grown grains and beans are the best choice.

Packaged Pastas ★★★

Nutritional Value: Fiber and B vitamins are still contained in most wheat pastas; the whole grain pastas have more fiber than the refined flour pastas. Enriched flour pastas will have additional B vitamins and possibly some iron added to them.
Cautions: These are usually made with refined wheat flour. Wheat is a common allergen.

Healthier Choices: Whole grain pastas and organic wheat pastas; also, there are wheat-free pastas made from rice, corn, or buckwheat.

Packaged Pasta Meals ★★★

Nutritional Value: This depends on the ingredients; there will be more nutrients if there are vegetables added. The pastas also contain fiber and some B-vitamins.

Cautions: These may be packaged with certain ingredients or additives that have potential risks, including MSG, salt, preservatives, animal fats, refined and enriched flour products, highly processed cheese additives, and food coloring in some of the macaroni and cheeses.

Healthier Choices: Fresh or home-cooked whole grain pastas with your own sauces or natural tomato sauces from jars.

Best Options: Organic whole grain pastas with tasty fresh sauces and toppings of tomatoes or other vegetables.

Pickles/Relishes ★★

Nutritional Value: Not very much nutrition in these since they are usually consumed in small quantities. However, there may be a few nutrients left from the little cucumbers that begin this food.

Cautions: Often treated with yellow dye #5 (listed) and sometimes highly sweetened with sugar or corn syrup. Also, there is concern with the salt content from the pickling process.

Healthier Choices: Brands without food coloring and lower sugar content.

Best Options: Organic pickles and relish, available in health food stores.

Fruit Juice Drinks ★★

Nutritional Value: These drinks may have a few nutrients not processed out from the fruits. Some may have added vitamin C and other fortified nutrients, otherwise they contain mostly fructose and calories.

Cautions: High-fructose corn syrup, sugar, and potentially harmful food colorings; many of the packaged drinks are made entirely with flavored high-fructose corn syrup (a concentrated sweetener). The low-calorie or imitation drinks may also contain aspartame and other artificial sweeteners and should be avoided or only consumed occasionally.

Healthier Choices: Naturally made fruit juice drinks or juice/mineral waters.

Best Options: Spring water, fresh juices in moderation, or regular mineral waters with your own added juice or herbal teabag. (Even at room temperature, this is a great drink.)

Fluid Replacement Drinks ★

Nutritional Value: These may have some added vitamins and minerals, such as sodium and potassium, to replace those lost from sweating.

Cautions: Food coloring, sugar, corn syrup, and glucose-fructose syrup, or the artificial sweetener aspartame. The disadvantages of the sweeteners and artificial colors outweigh the advantages of the minerals (electrolytes). The lift people feel is usually from the sugars.

Healthier Choices: Natural juice-sweetened fluid replacement drinks without added sugars and food coloring.

Best Options: Organic "thirst quenchers" or water with added electrolytes from products such as Emergen-C Lite.

Sodas ★

Nutritional Value: None, other than calories from added sugar or corn syrup. Diet sodas usually contain the artificial sweetener aspartame.

Cautions: High amounts of sugar or corn syrup, aspartame in diet drinks, caramel coloring and flavoring in colas, and artificial food colors in fruited or colored drinks. Try to limit you soda intake, especially those that are high in sugar and caffeine.

Healthier Choices: Natural sodas are available at both the health food store and supermarket.

Best Options: Spring water, herbal teas, and bottled herbal teas (but watch for added corn syrup).

Bottled Waters ★★★★

The cleanest product in the market—no calories, no fats, no sugar, just water. If you are going to drink bottled water on a regular basis, select brands bottled from a clean source (See Chapter 8).

Cautions: Source, chemicals, chlorine, and toxins from plastic bottles.

Coffee and Teas ★★

Nutritional Value: Limited nutrition, other than some nutrients contained in the herbal teas.
Cautions: Caffeine, pesticides, and other chemical contaminants from extraction processes.
Healthier Choices: If you want the caffeine, organic coffees and black teas have fewer chemicals; water-processed decafs are safer than those that are chemically processed.
Best Options: Herbal teas, organic if possible, and pure spring or filtered water.

Baby Foods ★★★

Nutritional Value: Baby foods will contain whatever nutrients that are available from the original foods that haven't been processed out. It is important to make sure that they provide supportive nutrition for your baby.
Cautions: Beware of nonorganic preparations, which often contain chemical pesticides; also watch for added sugars.
Healthier Choices: Brands such as Earth's Best and Tender Harvest are made with organic ingredients. Although they tend to be a bit more expensive, pesticide-free food is definitely better for your baby. At one store, a special on Tender Harvest made the price within two cents of the conventional, nonorganic brands. (See Chapter 7, for choices that are lower in pesticide residues.)
Best Options: You can prepare your own baby foods easily in the blender using appropriate organic ingredients. Simply blend portions of your own food using the 1-cup size jar for ease of handling.

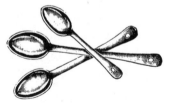

Gelatin Desserts ★

Nutritional Value: Very limited nutrition in these sugary products. Gelatin may have some value as a protein that supports nail and hair growth.
Cautions: Contains sugar and artificial colors; gelatin is mainly extracted from animal tissues
Healthier Choices: Make your own gelatin-type dessert from juice and gelatin, or even better, replace gelatin with the seaweed extract agar agar.

Jams and Jellies ★★

Nutritional Value: There may be some nutrients from the original fruits used to make these products; the more jamlike and less processed, the better, as in preserves or conserves.
Cautions: High sugar and fructose content, artificial coloring.
Healthier Choices: More natural and organic jams and jellies without added sugar, and made mostly of fruit. In any form, these should be used in moderation.

Peanut Butter ★★

Nutritional Value: Peanuts have a variety of nutrients, including niacin and other B vitamins, some minerals (depends on the soil in which they're grown), and essential oils.
Cautions: Hydrogenated oils/fats, overall fat content, sugar, salt, corn syrup, plus pesticides residues from treated peanuts; may also contain aflatoxin mold, which is a known carcinogen. Since even organic peanut butter can contain aflatoxins, try to alternate peanut products with other nuts and a variety of other foods.
Healthier Choices: Organic peanut butter, or other organic nut butters, such as almond or cashew butter, all in moderation. Some stores sell whole peanuts you can use to grind your own fresh peanut butter.

Salad Dressings ★★

Nutritional Value: Dressings provide fat calories from the oils used, some of which (healthy vegetable oils) are needed by our body for optimum functioning. Other nutrients may be present from other added ingredients.
Cautions: Fats, high in calories, preservatives, sugars, occasional food colorings.
Healthier Choices: All natural ingredients, cold-pressed vegetable oils, olive or canola oils—used in healthier brands without added sugars and preservatives.
Best Options: Make your own dressing with natural ingredients, fresh garlic, and other herbs.

Vegetable Oils ★★★

Nutritional Value: Vegetable oils contain some essential fatty acids that our bodies need to support tissues and cell membranes. Otherwise, they have few nutrients.
Cautions: Chemical and heat extraction processes used in production are a concern.
Healthier Choices: Naturally cold-pressed vegetable oils, extracted without heat or

chemicals; use a variety of polyunsaturated oils, such as corn, sunflower, or saf-flower, and monounsaturated oils, such as olive or canola oils. Polyunsaturates are best used unheated rather than in cooking because they break down easily when heated. The more stable monounsaturated oils can be used unheated or for cooking. **Best Options:** 1 to 2 tablespoons daily of organic, cold-pressed olive, canola or flax-seed oils

Soy Sauce and Tamari ★★

Nutritional Value: These fermented and salted soybean extracts have some nutrients from the soybeans and wheat from which they are extracted.
Cautions: High salt content, possible reactions for people with yeast problems or wheat sensitivities, and sodium benzoate as a mild preservative, which is generally well tolerated.
Healthier Choices: Low-sodium or wheat-free products, or nonfermented alternatives in the health food store (look at the labels).

Maple Syrups ★★★

Nutritional Value: Maple tree sap has a few nutrients, but is mostly simple sugar and calories. Artificial maple syrup is basically sugar or corn syrup, with caramel coloring and artificial flavors; there may be no trace of actual maple syrup in the product. Real maple syrup is actually extracted from a living tree.
Cautions: High sugar, high-fructose corn syrup, caramel coloring, aspartame in low-calorie syrups. Also, maple syrup made in America may contain formaldehyde contaminants, which still have not been banned in the extraction process. In Canada, the use of formaldehyde is not allowed.
Healthier Choices: Organic and formaldehyde-free pure maple syrups.

Tortillas ★★★★

Nutritional Value: Tortillas have some fiber, niacin, and other B vitamins from corn, and are sometimes soaked in lime, which adds calcium.
Cautions: May contain lard, some preservatives, and the new colored and flavored tortillas may contain artificial food coloring.
Healthier Choices: Although most tortillas are okay, better options are those made with whole grain, without preservatives, and made with organic flour or cornmeal.

Tortilla Chips ★★

Nutritional Value: Tortillas lose some of their value when they are fried to make chips and should be limited, primarily because of the fried oils.

Cautions: High fat content, especially excess hydrogenated fats, high salt content and lots of calories if you eat too many.

Healthier Choices: Chips made with organic corn, no hydrogenated oils.

Best Options: Only eat chips occasionally; instead try other snacks including fresh fruit or vegetables, or rice cakes with almond butter.

Breads ★★★

Nutritional Value: Breads can have decent nutritional value, especially when whole grains are used. Yet, often the refined flours are enriched and only fortified with some B vitamins and iron out of the original nutrients that have been lost in processing. Whole grain breads are also high in fiber, and may contain some minerals as well. It's hard to say anything bad about fresh baked bread because it's so good—and that's bad, because people tend to overconsume this delicious carbohydrate.

Cautions: Concerns include refined flours, preservatives, hydrogenated fats, sugars, and some people are sensitive to the higher yeast content or allergic to the wheat and gluten content.

Healthier Choices: Eat hearty whole grain breads without additives; for those with wheat or yeast allergies, there are also tasty wheat-free or yeast-free breads made from rice, millet, rye, or spelt flours.

Best Options: Eat more whole grains, such as rice and millet, instead of the baked grain flours. Also, substitute with organic rice cakes or corn tortillas. Some people are sensitive to the pesticide residues in whole wheat products and will tolerate organic products better. Thus, organic grain breads are the best option.

Crackers ★★★

Nutritional Value: Crackers contain dietary fiber and some vitamins and minerals, some of which are added back into the refined flour.

Cautions: Refined flours, hydrogenated fats, preservatives, salt, and sugars.

Healthier Choices: Whole grain crackers, or even better, organic wheat crackers with no additives. Since flavor and enjoyment of specific foods are mainly habits, there is value in shifting to healthier snacks for you and your children. See comments on Breads (above) for sensitivities to wheat.

Breakfast Cereals ★★

Nutritional Value: Most commercial cereals have limited nutrition, which is why they are also enriched and fortified with some B vitamins, calcium, iron, and sometimes other vitamins and minerals. Whole grain-based cereals have good amounts of dietary fiber.

Cautions: Excess sugar, food colorings, preservatives, and unlisted sulfites contained in dried fruits, such as raisins. Cereals are basically empty calories from refined grains (other than the added vitamins and minerals). Be sure to note the carbohydrate and fiber levels on the label. Also, there can be high amounts of artificial colorings in the rainbow-colored cereals, to which many children may be sensitive.

Healthier Choices: High-fiber, low calorie cereals like shredded wheat or bran cereals. Also, hot cereals such as oatmeal or cream of wheat have less added sugar. Unsweetened puffed cereals are also good. Some granolas are also wholesome, but brands with added dried fruit or nuts may have added sweeteners and be more highly caloric.

Best Options: Cooked organic whole grains, with fresh fruit, nuts, or seeds added, a sliced apple or banana and almonds or sunflower seeds.

Cookies ★★

Nutritional Value: Most of these are made from refined flour and sugar, and have minimal nutrition, unless enriched.

Cautions: High in fats and hydrogenated oils, excess sugar, refined wheat flour, and even coloring agents in the sugary decorations. Note that the serving size is often only 1 or 2 small cookies, which is hardly realistic. You may need to multiply the information to determine your calorie, carbohydrate, and fat intake.

Healthier Choices: There are cookies with less refined sugar, or sweetened with fruit juice; however, cookies should be in our treat food category and not part of our regular daily diet.

Best Options: Buy organic flour cookies with low added sugars, and eat as occasional treats.

Cake Mixes and Frostings ★

Nutritional Value: Like cookies, boxed cake mixes of refined flour and sugar provide few nutrients, unless enriched, and a little fiber.

Cautions: They usually contain refined flour and sugar with a variety of additives and preservatives. Cake mixes are primarily starch and sugar while the frostings are fat and sugar. Watch out for food colorings in any colorful frostings and decorations.

Healthier Choices: Some less refined choices are available with whole grain flours and less sugar.

Best Options: Homemade baked goods using primarily organic whole grain flours and other quality ingredients.

Fruit "Leathers" and Roll-Ups ★

Nutritional Value: These may have a few vitamins and minerals if they are made from fruit.

Cautions: Added sugar and food coloring, plus unlisted sulfites from the dried fruit component. This concentrated sweet can stick to your teeth and create a cavity risk.

Healthier Choices: More natural, and even organic fruit leathers, are available without added sugars and food coloring.

Best Options: Fresh fruit with less concentrated natural sugars.

Dairy Products (Milk and Cheese) ★★

Nutritional Value: Clearly, milk products have some nutritional value, including protein, calcium, phosphorus, and a variety of other minerals and vitamins.

Cautions: Whole milk is a concern because of the adverse effects of excess saturated fats in the diet; also, cow's milk is the most common food allergen in humans. Chemical contaminants from antibiotics, hormones, and many other drugs used in raising dairy cattle may be found in the milk and other dairy products we consume.

Healthier Choices: For milk-sensitive individuals, there are many tasty and healthy dairy substitutes that are based on soy or rice products; there are also many nonfat dairy and yogurt products, especially if you are watching your weight and fat intake. Likewise, there are low-fat cheeses, such as mozzarella and farmer's or hoop cheese.

Best Options: Organic dairy products; also, rotate milk products with milk substitutes.

Yogurt ★★★

Nutritional Value: With protein, calcium, and many other nutrients, yogurt can be very nutritious. Added fruits provide some additional nutrients, but these will add more sweeteners and calories.

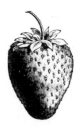

Cautions: May contain added sugars, corn syrup, or concentrated fruit as a sweetener, as well as food colorings, and high carbohydrate levels.

Healthier Choices: Low-fat and nonfat yogurts, yogurt that contains less than 25 grams of carbohydrate per serving. Remember, sweets and starches can cause weight gain, just as excess fats can.

Eggs ★★★

Nutritional Value: Eggs provide very good quality protein and a wide variety of vitamins and minerals, including B vitamins, calcium, magnesium, iron, and phosphorus.

Cautions: Chickens can pass on toxins from chemicals and pesticides in feeds, hormones to boost egg production, and antibiotic residues and other drugs from treatment for unsanitary, crowded conditions. Raw or undercooked eggs are a major source of salmonella infection. Also, egg allergy affects both adults and children.

Healthier Choices: You can buy eggs that come from free-range chickens that are fed better and cleaner food than those at the factory farms; egg cartons may also state "no antibiotics or preservatives used."

Best Options: Organic eggs are new to the market in some areas; chickens that are fed only organically-grown food can produce what are called organic eggs.

Mayonnaise ★

Nutritional Value: There is minimal food value in most mayonnaises other than some essential fatty acids contained in the vegetable oils, a few vitamins and minerals from lemon juice, and a little protein from the eggs.

Cautions: Mayonnaise should be eaten sparingly unless you are trying to gain weight or raise your blood fats. Once called "salad dressing," this is a high-fat food made with polyunsaturated oils, eggs, vinegars, sweeteners, and spices. Some contain emulsifiers and preservatives. Those watching their waistlines or who have an allergy to eggs should avoid mayonnaise.

Healthier Choices: Better quality mayos are now made with cold-pressed oils which are naturally extracted, and canola oil, which is a healthier monounsaturated fat. There are also lower-fat products available. Those that are made without preservatives and other food additives are an even better choice.

Weird Packaged Products (Are These Food?) ★

Artificial coffee creamers contain mainly hydrogenated oils and corn syrup; no actual food in these products.

Artificial whipped toppings are made from hydrogenated fats, sugars, chemicals, and not much else.

The Meat Counter—Meats, Fish, and Poultry

It is important to buy the freshest and cleanest animal meats as possible because animal proteins carry the highest risk with regard to microbial contamination. (Please refer to the information and charts in Chapter 9, *Food Preparation and Hygiene*, for proper storage and preparation of animal products and cooking temperatures necessary to eliminate your risk of foodborne infections from E. coli and other bacteria.)

Hamburger Meat ★★

Nutritional Value: Contains protein and a variety of nutrients like other beef foods.
Cautions: Watch out for the high fat levels. Because hamburger is ground up, it can have just about anything in it, including the lower quality cuts or higher amounts of fat. Also, the chemicals used in cattle often end up in heavier concentration in the fats.
Healthier Choices: Ground turkey meat is a popular replacement for hamburger beef. There are also very good soy and grain burgers available in most stores. I particularly enjoy tofu burgers that have small cut-up vegetables in them. Melt some good cheese on your "burger," place it on a wholesome bun or bread, and cover it with some ketchup, pickles, onion, tomato, lettuce, or whatever you like.

Steaks and Other Beef Cuts ★★

Nutritional Value: Cattle muscle, which is basically what a steak is, usually has a fair amount of nutrition. Besides a high amount of protein, beef contains many B vitamins and a wide variety of minerals, especially hard-to-obtain iron and zinc. The fat content also can be relatively low, and you can trim much of it before you cook your cut.
Cautions: Animal muscle can also hold whatever toxins the animal has been exposed to, as well as the toxins that it creates when it is slaughtered. Livestock chemical exposure is probably of more concern than any other food (see Chapters 2 and 3).

Healthier Choices: There are many animal and vegetable alternatives to beef that will also provide quality protein and nutrients. These include fish, poultry, and legumes.

Chicken and Turkey ★★★

Nutritional Value: Chicken and turkey provide some important nutrition, including quality protein and a wide variety of vitamins and minerals, such as B vitamins, calcium, magnesium, iron, and phosphorus. Turkey is also known to contain a high amount of tryptophan, an amino acid that supports serotonin, which has positive effects on our moods and sleep.

Cautions: Poultry products can pass on toxins from chemicals and pesticides in feeds, hormones to boost size, plus antibiotics and other drugs from treatment for unsanitary, crowded conditions so common in the large factory farms. Chicken can also pass on many microbes if it is not cleaned or cooked adequately.

Healthier Choices: Free-range chickens that are allowed to forage for their feed are usually healthier birds and a better quality food.

Pork ★★

Nutritional Value: Pork also provides high-quality protein and a variety of minerals and B vitamins. Most of the cuts, other than the lunchmeats made from pork, are fairly low in fat.

Cautions: This "other white meat," as it has been advertised by the pork producers, should not be classified with poultry instead of beef. Chemical exposure and potential microbes are a minor concern nowadays, since trichinosis seems to have been nearly eliminated. But pork is most often consumed in the form of bacon, ham, and other lunchmeats, which often have higher fat levels and are preserved with salt and nitrites.

Healthier Choices: Again, other protein sources include poultry, seafood, and vegetable-based proteins.

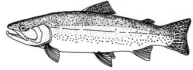

Seafood ★★★

Nutritional Value: Saltwater and freshwater fish are considered by many to be some of the most nutritious food available. High in protein with good amounts of many vitamins and minerals, including iron, iodine, and zinc, many fish also contain healthful oils such as the omega-3s—EPA and DHA.

Cautions: Fish may contain excess mercury from ocean contamination; swordfish and tuna are particularly suspect, but any fish can carry toxic metals from the surrounding waters. Since so many lakes and rivers in our country continue to be polluted by industry and agriculture, we may be exposed to a wide variety of chemical toxins, including sewage and industrial solvents, and pesticide runoff from freshwater species. And we may want to avoid coastal fish like cod or red snapper, and many shellfish, which filter garbage and toxins from the sea (see below).

Healthier Choices: If we choose to eat seafood regularly, we should vary, or rotate, our choices so that we minimize specific chemical or toxic metal accumulation. Deep sea fish like halibut, sea bass, and sole may be less exposed and thus, cleaner of chemicals. These can be rotated into the diet as well. Pond-raised fish, such as trout, are not exposed to the wide array of chemicals in our oceans.

Shellfish ★

Shellfish include the hard-shelled mollusks: clams, oysters, mussels, and scallops—and the softer-shelled crustaceans: crabs, shrimp, and lobsters.

Nutritional Value: With protein, good fats, and loads of vitamins and minerals, these foods can be quite nutritious. The mollusks tend to contain higher amounts of zinc and copper than any other known foods.

Cautions: Because shellfish both breathe (and many feed) by filtering seawater through their bodies, and they live, generally, in more heavily polluted coastal waters, toxins seem to accumulate and remain in their tissues in greater concentration than in any other seafood. This may contribute to the fact that more people are allergic to or get sick more often from shellfish than to other kinds of seafood.

Healthier Choices: I think that shrimp and crab are nutritious foods, to be eaten occasionally by those who aren't allergic. Clams and oysters are riskier in terms of microbial and chemical contamination, and they should be rare treats during safe months; some find these foods rather aphrodiasical. Most other seafood, other animal proteins, and vegetarian proteins are good substitutes for shellfish. As stated before, seafood should be varied to reduce repetitive exposure to the same toxins, which provides greater risk for food poisoning.

Bacon, Hot Dogs, Lunchmeats ★

Nutritional Value: These may contain some protein and nutrients depending on the cuts of meat used and the production process.

Cautions: Watch for the carcinogenic nitrites, as well as high fats and sodium. Also, very low-quality meat or non-meat products are used in some brands. This category should be avoided or only eaten occasionally.

Healthier Choices: Oven-roasted turkey and any nitrite-free, low-fat poultry cuts. There are hot dogs, some cold-cuts, including pastrami and bologna, and even bacon, made from soybeans and/or grains and vegetables. They are naturally seasoned without chemicals and very flavorful, and often smell and taste much like the "real thing."

Deli Products ★★

Nutritional Value: This will obviously depend on what products you buy, and this can range from very nutritious contents to high-fat, high-calorie, non-nutritious items.

Cautions: Fats and mayonnaise, frying oils, salt, added sugar in many products and possible contamination in leftovers or aged foods; deli products are subject to airborne bacteria. Be a bit wary of prepared items because they are usually not labeled, so we don't really know what's in them, i.e., their fat or sugar content, calorie count, etc.

Healthier Choices: Ask about the ingredients in dishes that interest you and make sure they are fresh; stay away from items with eggs or shellfish.

Best Options: Make your own potato salad, or other dishes, at home using fresh ingredients.

Tofu and Other Soy Products ★★★★

Nutritional Value: Tofu and all soy products contain good quality protein and fatty acids from the soybeans, from which they are made. They also have many vitamins and minerals, including calcium. Soybean products appear to have estrogenic activity and may br helpful for women as they age and enter menopause.

Cautions: Soy products are basically healthy foods, however, tofu does have over 25% fat calories, even though these are healthy vegetable oils. Also, some people are allergic to soybeans and tofu.

Healthier Choices: Make a grain and vegetable dish with tofu as a meal; it is very satisfying and highly nutritious, healthy choice. There are also other soy products, especially tempeh, which are fermented soy bean cakes. For people avoiding cow's milk products, there are soy-based frozen desserts, soy cheese, and soy yogurts, which are all very tasty.

Frozen Foods ★★

There is a wide array of frozen products, including vegetables, pizzas, waffles, desserts, juices, and even entire meals. Although there are some good values here, you will often pay more for the extra costs of creating and maintaining frozen foods. Meat and produce that are frozen fresh appear to retain the highest level of nutrition, second only to foods that are Nature-fresh. However, be aware of a wide variety of food additives in standard frozen foods.

Ice Cream ★

Nutritional Value: Most ice creams contain lots of calories, good for people trying to gain weight. The milk content also provides some protein and calcium, and other milk-based nutrients.

Cautions: Very high fat and high sugar, excessive calories, food colorings in most colored ice creams, preservatives, emulsifiers, milk allergens; regard this food as an occasional treat only.

Healthier Choices: Ice cream made from natural ingredients, low-fat ice creams, natural colors or no added colors, nondairy ice creams made from soybeans or rice.

Best Options: Fruit sorbets, fruit smoothies, nonfat plain yogurt with fruit, Dr. Elson's nice cream (frozen fruit run through a Champion juicer), which is frosty and creamy and absolutely free of milk and fat!

Frozen Dinners ★★

Nutritional Value: Depending on what you buy, these can contain protein from animal-based foods, fiber from grains, and other nutrients from vegetable-based foods.

Cautions: Saturated fats, hydrogenated fats in fried foods, added salt and sugar, and a long list of additives.

Healthier Choices: Healthy versions of TV dinners with good animal protein selections, fresh frozen veggies, and a minimum of additives.

Best Options: Make your own fresh and wholesome meals at home. If time is an issue, try preparing a number of meals all in one day and freeze for later use.

Frozen Pizzas ★★

Nutritional Value: These will have some fiber and B vitamins from the pizza crust, some vitamins C and beta-carotene from the tomato sauce, calcium and protein from the cheese, and more protein and other nutrients from added meats or vegetables, such as olives, mushrooms, peppers, etc.

Cautions: High-fat cheeses, nitrites and other chemicals in meats (pepperoni and sausage), preservatives, and dough conditioners.

Healthier Choices: Frozen veggie pizzas with less cheese and extra tomato sauce; homemade with store-bought crusts, healthy tomato sauce, mozzarella cheese, black olives, garlic, sliced tomatoes, etc. Pizza can provide a fairly balanced meal (especially if you add some vegetables) for kids who may not otherwise make many healthy food choices.

Best Options: Organic ingredients—wheat, dairy, and veggies.

Frozen French Fries ★★

Nutritional Value: These have minimal nutrition, but some fiber from the potatoes. A few brands contain some enriched nutrients.

Cautions: Hydrogenated and heated oils, sulfites, polyunsaturated fats, sugars, and preservatives.

Healthier Choices: Natural and organic french fries using good quality oils, such as canola.

Best Options: Baked "fries" are absolutely delicious. Cut up your own potatoes (organic ones if possible) at home and bake them on a cookie sheet in the oven. Do a light slather with olive oil and sprinkle with a little veggie salt before you bake. Serve with a natural ketchup.

Frozen Juices and Drinks ★★

Nutritional Value: Very similar to fruit juice drinks, they have some nutrients from the original fruits from which the juice is made, but much of the nutrition is lost with processing. Some have added vitamin C and other vitamins or minerals, such as calcium or iron.

Cautions: Added sugars, food colorings, and any hidden chemicals from growing, harvesting, storing, and extracting the concentrates.

Healthier Choices: Pure fruit juices without the added sweeteners or colorings.

Best Options: Organic frozen juices, or squeeze your own at home, buy them freshly squeezed, or simply get in the habit of eating whole fruit instead.

Fresh Produce ★★★★

Nutritional Value: These are the most nutritious foods in the store. Each fruit and vegetable contains its own specific mix of vitamins and minerals, so eating a variety is best.

Cautions: Primary concerns are chemical contamination, as discussed in Chapters 2 and 3, as well as produce that is known to be more heavily treated with pesticides, such as strawberries (see Chapter 7).

Best Options: Buy organically grown produce whenever possible.

The Natural Food Stores

The natural food industry has grown by leaps and bounds over the past two decades, and especially in the 1990s. Overall, it is providing products that are made with more attention to nutrition, and with a minimum of synthetic chemicals. Ideally, these are "foods from Nature" or at least closer to Nature. There are innovative products to use as healthier replacements for milk, such as soy milk and rice milks or amazake (a sweet rice drink), as well as basic products that have been improved, including organic whole wheat breads, organic corn chips cooked in cold-pressed, monounsaturated oils (instead of hydrogenated fats), and more wholesome soups, pasta sauces, macaroni and cheese, and a hundred other items. Just about any of the processed foods found in the supermarket has comparative products in the natural food store. Although by and large, you won't find products with artificial food coloring, nitrites, or lard, or much hydrogenated fats, there are some cautions.

Cautions: Many high-fat, high-sugar foods, such as ice creams, chips, cookies, and crackers, that are available in health food stores should not be a very significant part of your diet. You still need to focus on purchasing and consuming mainly fresh fruits and vegetables, whole grains and legumes, and other nutritious, less processed foods.

The natural food store is usually a bit more expensive than the typical grocery store. However, most are competitive and offer many specials and good values. You still will pay more for organic produce. If creating your own garden or greenhouse is not possible, I believe we should be willing to pay a little more for better quality, fresher produce that offers few (if any) chemicals and the best possible nutrition.

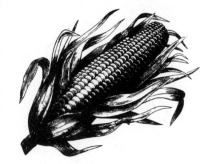

CHAPTER SEVEN

Organic Foods: Why, When, and What to Buy

♦

The negative impact of treating the Earth with chemicals, of spraying the fields and the orchards, reaches beyond any food product. It affects the surrounding land, air, water, people, and animals—even the ozone layer—as well as those who consume the food. The regular consumption of chemicals from foods causes a variety of health problems, the worst being cancer and the pain and suffering that accompanies it. In addition, there are other immune, neurologic, cognitive, and hormonal effects of chemical and pesticide exposure.

Chemical agricultural "warfare" has clearly gotten out of hand. In 1995, the United States alone used more than 270 billion pounds of artificial fertilizers and 2 billion pounds of pesticides. For the last twenty years, the U.S. agricultural industry has used more than 1 billion pounds of pesticides annually. This lack of concern, and often unconscious behavior, has generated the organic farming movement—growing, harvesting, and shipping safer foods for public consumption without the use of chemicals—as a tangible statement of gratitude for the gift of life from Mother Nature.

ORGANIC FARMING

Organic farming means growing foods without using chemicals on the soil, on plants, or on the harvested product. The growth and current success of organic farming in this country demonstrates the public's growing awareness of health and environmental issues and its desire for safer food. The organic farming sector has grown from a modest enterprise made up of small farming networks with gross sales of $78 million in 1980 to an agricultural industry with sales of more than $4 billion in 1997. This industry has grown nearly 50% every year for the past seven years. Three out of every ten consumers are now buying organically grown produce. Also, in an interview of general consumers by *Prevention* magazine, over 50% stated they would purchase organic foods if there was a national standard.

REASONS TO BUY ORGANIC FOODS

- Prevent health problems caused by toxic chemicals
- Enjoy foods with the highest possible nutrition
- Enjoy more flavorful food
- Protect future generations from chemical pollution
- Decrease the real cost of food, by not supporting the use of chemicals
- Decrease the cost of organic food by increasing demand
- Help independent farmers
- Prevent soil contamination and erosion
- Protect water quality
- Reduce ozone damage to the atmosphere
- Restore biodiversity, protecting animal and plant life
- Protect future generations from chemical pollution

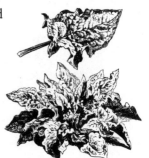

All across America, organic farming is making modest but real inroads into mainstream agriculture. In the northeast, 70% of the apple growers are exploring alternative (organic) practices. In the vineyards from the northwest to the northeast, growers are minimizing their use of chemicals on the fields and in production, using more natural substances to process wines and using steam to sterilize equipment rather than chemicals.

In California, many farms are successfully using the organic approach in the cultivation of produce, in orchards, vineyards, and even on poultry farms. Although organic agriculture takes place on a smaller scale than mainstream agribusiness, organic farmers are growing a wide range of crops from lettuces and squashes to melons and wine grapes. Size becomes an advantage: organic farms and nurseries can specialize, and have been noted to raise more than a hundred varieties of apples and thirty kinds of pears on one farm. In addition to economic success, organic farmers express satisfaction in that they are restoring the land, farming in a way that will not harm wildlife or humans, all while raising healthy crops.

Community supported agriculture (CSA) is another aspect of the expanding organics movement. In 1997 there were at least 500 CSAs in the United States. This is a cooperative arrangement in which the farmers agree to provide produce if a number of families or a community make a contractual commitment to support the farm. This results in the reliable delivery of primarily chemical-free, fresh produce each week in the summer and root vegetables regularly in the autumn and winter.

What Exactly Is Organic Farming?

The basis of organic farming involves the use of the least chemical, most natural methods of pest and weed control; it also means using the most natural, least chemical methods for developing and supporting nutrient-rich soil. The philosophy is that healthy soil leads to healthy crops. Many of these agricultural practices have been developed and used all over the world for thousands of years, and have come back into favor as a "postmodern" phenomenon. In California and some other states, there are legal guidelines that stipulate the kinds of practices a farm must follow in order to label its produce "organic."

Some of the regulations for growing organically include:

1. No use of chemicals in the growing areas or in the 25-foot "buffer zones" around fields, which protects them from spray or chemical drift.

   In California, one of the few states that have legislated certified organic standards, crops cannot be considered officially organic—grown without toxic chemicals—until no chemicals have been used for three years. Even then, these foods may still contain traces of long-lived chemicals. For this reason, organic standards provide for maximum levels of possible contaminants.

2. No use of sewer sludge as fertilizer in any part of the growing process. Sewer sludge contains a variety of chemicals, toxins and microbes.

   Reports from the National Sludge Alliance (based on EPA reports of 1989) suggest that sewer sludge contains potentially 60,000 different toxic chemicals that include residential and industrial byproducts, hospital wastes, toxic metals, pesticides, solvents, and radioactive wastes, as well as 25 potentially infectious agents that include the salmonella and E. coli bacteria, and hepatitis A virus.

3. Specific rules for feeding, housing, and medically treating any livestock that generate food. This includes clear guidelines to minimize the use of antibiotics in these animals.

   Goals for ecologically sound husbandry include raising hormone-free livestock, limiting the use of antibiotics and other drugs to cases of illness, and prohibiting the feeding of ground-up animal parts.

4. Specific regulations for the amount and kind of chemicals used in food-processing plants for packaging of organic foods, including the types of cleansers and disinfectants.

   Toxic chemicals, such as solvents or any potentially carcinogenic compounds, are not to be used in areas that come in contact with food or with equipment that may contaminate the food.

In order to have their products certified as organic in California, growers undergo farm inspection, including the analysis of their soil's nutrient content. They must document all crop and soil inputs, and develop soil fertility and pest control plans. In addition, they are required to keep complete yield, harvest, and sales records, undergo at least two inspections before they can be certified, and have yearly inspections after that.

Aside from these legal requirements that form the basis for organic certification, the fundamentals of organic farming integrate ecological principles into farming practices. While organic farming can't ensure that products are totally free of residues, the methods used minimize pollution to the soil, air, and water. Organic systems rely on crop rotation, animal and plant manures, mechanical cultivation, and biological pest management to enrich the soil and control insect infestations and weeds through the least invasive means (Certified California Organic Farmers).

Produce listed as "pesticide free" may lack the advantages of the above comprehensive approach to farming. "Pesticide free" simply means that the edible parts of a crop haven't been sprayed, but it could still be raised with synthetic fertilizers, insecticides, and fungicides. "Residue free" means that a lab analysis found no specific residues on a particular food, but testing usually focuses only on certain chemicals among the more than 870 registered pesticides. Tests are performed at random, and there is no assurance that the producer has a commitment to building the soil or avoiding the use of synthetic chemicals. Neither of these

ESSENTIALS OF ORGANIC GROWING

Develop Healthy Soil	Composting; animal manures; green manure crops (e.g.. alfalfa) that are plowed back into the soil for nourishment; rock powders, gypsum, and lime for mineral content; encourage earthworms, which aerate the soil, prevent compaction, and release nutrients
Use Crop Rotation	Helps rest the soil, and control plant diseases; limit insect populations; condition the soil; maintain nutrient-rich soil
Intercrop Planting	Integrate planting of food crops with ground covers, including flowering plants that attract beneficial insects
Use of Cover Crops	Act like mulch, to hold moisture, secure the soil against erosion from wind and rain; add nitrogen to the soil; discourage pest populations; minimize the use of herbicides and fumigants; reduce harmful high salt or nitrate content
Healthy Cultivation Practices	To minimize herbicides, remove weeds with a cultivator such as the French plow, which trims between the rows
Integrated Pest Management	Uses a systems strategy to control pests, with least-toxic chemicals as a last resort Identify pests and their natural enemies Monitor and record levels of pest populations Determine damage, match treatment to problem Factor in environmental variables, such as weather Apply effective methods that are the least disruptive
Sustainable Plant Production	Analyze the farming environment Select plant species and varieties appropriate to the farm environment Diversify crops and agriculture methods Manage soil quality Humane approach to both wildlife and animal husbandry
Use of Natural Enemies to Control Pest Populations	Maintain a balance between different pest populations Encourage the natural enemies of harmful insects, such as spiders, ladybugs, lace wings, flies, wasps and hornets, predatory mites, insect-feeding birds

terms have a legal definition, and appear to be used more for marketing when the producer or seller cannot use "organic." However, when we buy food that is labeled "organic," we can be assured that the practices listed on page 109 have been followed. In addition, when we buy organic food we show our support for the continued growth of the organic movement and the standards set forth by such groups as the Certified California Organic Farmers (CCOF). Our purchase of organic foods encourages the development of similar national standards for raising food without chemical contamination.

How Costly and How Available Is Organic Food?

The cost of organic products is often higher than the same nonorganic fruit, vegetable, or grain because of the smaller size of the average farm and the additional labor involved. Understandably, many are unwilling to pay the extra money unless they have experienced adverse affects of chemical exposure or the benefits of a chemical-free diet. Once you experience the health benefits of eating the most wholesome food available, as I have in both my medical practice and in my own life, you will come to realize that feeling better is well worth a few extra dollars out of your weekly grocery budget as a preventive health investment.

In recent years, organic foods have become more plentiful and of higher quality, and some are now available at a lower cost. More and more shoppers are finding that the taste and the reassurance of quality nutrition and chemical avoidance make buying organic worthwhile. Many supermarkets offer a choice between nonorganic and organic, so consumers have an ongoing opportunity to see and taste the difference. Mail-order catalogs (many found on the Internet) also provide a way to make organic food and other products accessible to more people. This movement is clearly spreading and this suggests an important trend for the future.

Eating Out Organic

An exciting and healthy trend in dining out is that many restaurants, especially those in larger cities, are now featuring organic foods. Thriving establishments with this wholesome approach include Chez Panisse in Berkeley, Greens and Millenium in San Francisco, Nora's in Washington, DC, and Moosewood in upstate New York. Locally grown fresh produce, tropical foods, and specialty crops have become a major attraction as well. And as the chefs become increasingly committed to buying

FIVE HEALTH BENEFITS OF ORGANIC FOODS

1. Crops grown in the rich soil of organic farms appear to have higher nutrient values than nonorganic produce. A study done at Doctor's Data lab in Chicago, and published in the *Journal of Applied Nutrition* (Vol. 45, 1993), compared organic produce with similar conventionally grown fruits and vegetables. They found that on average the organic pears, apples, potatoes, sweet corn, and wheat had over 90% more vitamins and minerals than similar commercial food—almost twice the nutrient content!

2. Organic foods have minimal toxicity and therefore place less chemical burden on the body, especially on the liver, the immune system, the brain, and the nervous system. At least half of the most frequently used agricultural chemicals are nerve toxins and can cause irritation and overstimulation of the nervous system.

3. The risk of disease is reduced—particularly for degenerative conditions such as cancer, and for conditions, such as allergies and hyperactivity, which may be brought on by reactions to chemicals.

4. Overall health is enhanced by the consumption of these more wholesome foods.

5. The local environmental pollution is reduced—by avoiding pesticidal sprays and gases, there is no chemical runoff to surrounding lands, the local water supply, and less air pollution. This is a sensible way to protect Nature, the animals and neighboring humans.

Example: One case of a clear health benefit from eating organic food has been provided by a recent Danish study, which found that men who consumed a diet composed of at least 25% organic produce had sperm counts 43% higher than those who ate conventional foods.

organic foods and supporting local growers (and some even have their own gardens), this movement will continue to expand.

Sampling organic food when you eat out is a great way to become acquainted with the excellent flavor of produce grown in rich soil without the use of pesticides. And it's a good way to inspire yourself to use this healthy approach in your own cooking.

WHICH FOODS ARE MOST IMPORTANT TO BUY ORGANICALLY GROWN?

There are certain key foods that are more important to buy organically grown, because some crops are more heavily treated than others. Of produce grown in the U.S., as much as 70% has been found by the FDA to have some pesticide residues. More than half of everything we usually eat introduces some pesticides into our body. However, no existing research that has looked into the long-term effects of small doses of thousands of different chemicals over a lifetime. What we have learned from countless of research studies on people who work on farms and in

TWENTY-FIVE FOODS TO BUY ORGANIC

Product	Concern
Baby Foods	Possible effects of neurotoxins on developing infant
Milk and butter	Pesticides are stored in fats and can be passed on to us
Fruits	
Strawberries	70% had residues, highest content of endocrine-disrupters; on average, 300 pounds of pesticides per acre
Bananas	Baby's first food; banana sprays highly toxic
Peaches, Cherries, Nectarine, Apricots	About 70% of each of these stone fruits had residues
Apples	Contain a large number of different pesticides
Grapes	79% of grapes tested from Chile had residues
Melons	Mexican cantaloupe: 76% residues; Honeydew: 69% residues
Red raspberries	56% had residues; 31% had 5 different residues
Imported produce	Sprays used that are banned in the U.S.; buy U.S. produce in season
Vegetables	
Bell Peppers	64% had residues, highest level of neurotoxins
Leafy Greens—Lettuces	Treated with systemic pesticides that cannot be washed off
Spinach	Systemic pesticides; most carcinogens, most endocrine-disrupters

pesticide manufacturing is that very real adverse health effects are linked to the use of pesticides.

With this risk from chemical exposure, it makes sense to choose organic foods. Since there is no labeling that discloses chemicals used in growing, storing, or shipping, we don't know what was done by each farmer to each crop. Thus, we can't really make an informed choice—yet.

Having reviewed the most relevant research on pesticides and additives in food, I have come up with the following list of **25 Important Foods to Buy Organically Grown**. They are listed in an order from what I consider the highest level of health risk.

Vegetables *continued*

Green beans	Heavily treated, most sprays are systemic, endocrine-disrupters
Tomatoes	On some samples, 30 different pesticides found
Cucumbers	Second highest level of carcinogenic pesticides

Grains

Rice	Conventional fields heavily treated
Corn	Corn receives an excessive amount of U.S. pesticides
Oats	Also may be overtreated
Whole wheat	More than 90% of all wheat samples had pesticides (FDA)

Protein Foods

Eggs	Factory farming increases bacteria, decreases quality
Seafood	Many rivers and estuaries polluted; important to know source
Meats	Animals often raised with hormones, antibiotics, other drugs

Beverages

Coffee	Sprays aren't always burned off in roasting
Wine	Grapes and wines frequently treated with chemicals and sulfites (which can be allergenic)

Source: Data integrated from the Environmental Working Group, Center for Science in the Public Interest, and *E Magazine*.

---

1. Baby Foods: Since infants are more sensitive to pesticides because of their more vulnerable nervous and immune systems, organic baby foods are much safer. Unless you specifically buy organic, studies show that your baby may be getting toxic chemicals in common foods such as green beans and applesauce. Fortunately, there are several companies marketing organic baby foods in mainstream grocery stores. Or, even better, make your own fresh baby food in the blender from organic fruits and vegetables.

2. Strawberries: This is the most heavily contaminated produce item in the U.S. today, according to data from a number of environmental groups, including a 1993 study by the Environmental Working Group (Washington, DC) and an analysis by the Pesticide Action Network (PANNA). Strawberries in California are treated with more than 300 pounds of pesticides per acre, and some areas of the country use up to 500 pounds per acre. As a comparison, conventional farm-ing currently uses 25 pounds of pesticides per acre on the aver-age crop. Also, some growers may be spraying the harvested strawberries for shipping. This adds to the amount of chemi-cal concentration in the fruit. Strawberries were also found to have the highest level of hormone-affecting pesticides, includ-ing benomyl, vinclozolin, and endosulfan. Methyl bromide is another common spray used on strawberries. Note that out-of-season strawberries may be most heavily treated because they come from other countries and are sprayed even more before shipping.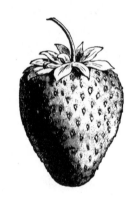

3. Milk and Butter: Because pesticides are pervasive and stored in higher amounts in the fat, dairy products tend to retain higher levels of residues and chemicals from feeds and other sources. This is not well researched yet; however, it makes total sense to me, and therefore my family with growing children is buying organic milk products. Milk is a common source of the herbicide atrazine (a known endocrine-disrupter) and the growth hormone BGH, which has been genetically engineered to boost milk production. Almost 80% of the cows treated with BGH get udder infec-tions, so there is also increased risk of antibiotics in the milk. These concerns have motivated shoppers to consider organic milk products more seriously, and the sale of organic milk is now averaging $50 to $60 million each year. It is becoming more available in mainstream supermarkets.

4. Bananas: If you are mashing bananas for babies or feeding them frequently to the kids, buy them organic whenever possible. Because they are shipped from southern and tropical countries, and they are exposed to some chemicals at all phases of growth and production, they may be receiving heavier pesticide exposure. Bananas are commonly gassed with ethylene (even some organics) to ripen them and prepare them for shipping, and this seems to be relatively nontoxic to the banana consumer. They are also being fumigated with ethyl bromide to prevent pests from coming in with the fruit. I am most concerned about this exposure, and so I buy organic bananas, which are more available these days. Although the studies suggest that much of the contamination can be peeled off, organic bananas are the safest option for children.

5. Stone Fruits (Peaches, Cherries, Apricots, Plums, and Nectarines): Stone fruits are often sprayed to protect them because their sweetness attracts many insects. They are often sprayed after they are packed into boxes for shipping. Since their skins are very absorptive, they tend to retain more of the chemicals. In FDA spot checks, 71% of the peach crops had pesticide residues, and peach farms also tended to have one of the highest rates of pesticide violations. Cherries are another heavily sprayed crop; the FDA found more pesticide residues on U.S. cherries than they did on the imported ones. Apricots frequently had residues (64%), and 35% had the carcinogenic pesticide captan present.

6. Leafy Greens (Lettuces, Spinach, Kale, and Chard): Sprayed chemicals tend to remain on the leaves of these vegetables, which is potentially more harmful since we eat the leafy parts. In FDA studies, spinach was the leafy green most frequently found to contain the more potent pesticides, especially the organophosphates (neurotoxins) and permethrin (noted as mildly carcino-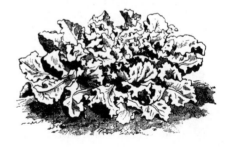genic). In addition, 10% of the spinach samples had residues of DDT, which was phased out of use in the U.S. over 25 years ago.

7. Grapes: Unless they are organically grown, grapes may receive multiple applications of a variety of chemical agents during their growing period. Some fruits and vegetables are more highly sensitive to the environment, particularly those that ripen quickly or attract insects and molds. These crops, including grapes, tend to be more heavily treated in order to get them to the market (and to protect the financial interest of the grower). FDA research indicates that imported grapes are even more heavily treated than the U.S. samples. During winter and early spring, almost all grapes available in the U.S. are from Chile, and these are found to have an exceptionally high percentage of pesticide residues (79%). They also have a higher percent of the carcinogenic pesticides, captan and iprodione. However, U.S. grape growers use high amounts of sulfites and the fumigant, methyl bromide, so these are all good reasons to buy organic grapes and grape juices.

8. Green Beans: Consider buying your green beans organically grown because the EPA has registered more than 60 pesticides in use on green beans, and the FDA found 23 different chemicals on green beans in its 1992–1993 studies. Additionally, almost 10% of the imported green beans contained illegal pesticide residues.

9. Apples: A staple in many diets, apples have been found to be nearly as contaminated as strawberries. Forty-eight different pesticides were detected by FDA testing in nearly 2,500 samples from 1984 to 1991, while 36 different chemicals were found in their 1992–1993 evaluations. Nearly half of these chemicals were either neurotoxic or carcinogenic. In the FDA analyses, apples and peaches had 7 different pesticides per crop. Fortunately, a shift away from spraying the orchards is 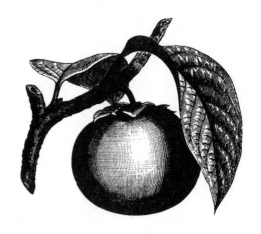 occurring in some areas. As mentioned earlier, 70% of the apple growers in the Northeast are using organic practices and integrated pest management, an intermediary process towards organic that involves the use of helpful insects to control more destructive ones. If you buy nonorganic apples, be sure to peel them and discard the skin before you eat them since most of the chemical residues are on the apple skins. It's time to change our saying to "an organic apple a day keeps the doctor away."

10. Rice: This is the most frequently consumed food on the planet. You should seriously consider buying organically grown rice and rice products, especially if it is one of your staple foods. The dangerous herbicide 2,4,5-T was sprayed on rice before it was banned in 1984, and many persistent water-soluble herbicides and insecticides have been found to contaminate the ground water near major rice fields, such as in California's Sacramento River Valley. I suggest buying organic rice in bulk. You'll find that this way it's as economical as nonorganic prepackaged rice and much safer.

11. Corn Products: A primary staple in the American diet, corn is typically heavily treated; nearly 50% of all pesticides are sprayed on corn. Locally grown fresh corn tends to be treated less, so sweet corn on the cob is likely safer than corn byproducts, which may have more contamination. However, corn is still heavily treated with the herbicide atrazine and it is also typically sprayed after harvesting.

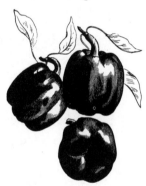

12. Sweet Peppers: Both red and green bell peppers were found to have many chemical residues from the most neurotoxic of the pesticides. In the FDA's measurement of both U.S. and Mexican crops, 64% of peppers contained at least 1 pesticide, while 36% contained 2 or more. These vegetables also may be waxed, which makes it difficult to remove the residues and other chemicals within the waxes.

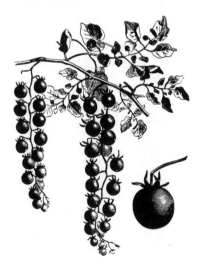

13. Tomatoes: One study found that as many as 30 different pesticides are used to spray tomatoes. Because the skins of tomatoes are thin and absorbent, and since this is a staple in many salads, soups, and sauces, tomatoes are worth buying organically grown. At certain times of year, the price of organic plum tomatoes is competitive with nonorganic varieties. Farmer's markets may be the best source of all for fresh unsprayed tomatoes. Or they can be easily grown on a deck or in planter boxes at home.

14. Tropical Fruits: Pineapples, papayas, and mangoes are very attractive to tropical pests and may be more heavily treated during cultivation, preparation, and shipping. Because of their thin skins, they tend to absorb the sprays, creating higher levels of chemical contamination. We call these systemic pesticides, and they cannot be washed away as they are contained within the fruit and seeds.

15. Celery : Although most people do not eat a lot of celery all at once, it can be an ideal, low-calorie snack food. This very absorptive, watery vegetable understandably retains residues, so it is not surprising that on EPA analyses, 81% of samples contained residues, more pesticides than any other crop. Furthermore, many of the pesticides found were the stronger neurotoxic and carcinogenic ones. After reading this report, I added celery to my list of important foods to buy organically grown.

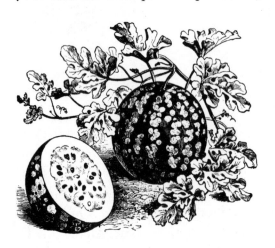

16. Berries (Raspberries, Blueberries, Blackberries): As with strawberries, these berries have high pesticide exposure during cultivation, and most of these are systemic, meaning they get into the fruit. Over 50% of EPA- tested raspberries had pesticide residues, and nearly a third had 2 or more. It is best to find your own untreated patch to pick from, or buy them organically grown.

17. Imported Produce: This usually out-of-season produce is often heavily treated for easier growing and shipping to the United States. There is also risk of higher toxicity from the use of chemicals that have been banned in America. Cantaloupes and other imported melons were found to have a high concentration of pesticides in two thirds of tested samples. In Mexican cantaloupes, 48% had 2 or more residues.

18. Cruciferous Vegetables (Broccoli, Cabbage, Brussels Sprouts, and Cauliflower): Because of their healthy, anticancer nutrient content, high fiber, and low calories, these are excellent foods to eat regularly. But since we eat the parts that may have been sprayed with carcinogenic chemicals, it's best to eat the organically grown versions of these vegetables.

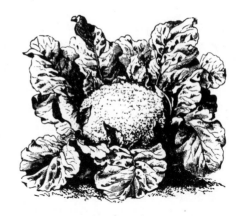

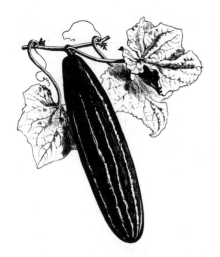

19. Cucumbers: These appear on Earth Working Group's "buy organic" list because of the potent pesticide, dieldrin, found in nonorganic cucumber crops. Dieldrin increases cancer risk. Also, the waxes commonly used to make cucumbers shiny should be avoided because they may contain other chemical residues.

20. Wheat: Many grains and legumes, particularly wheat, rice, and corn, are treated with pesticides as crops and then fumigated periodically during storage. In a recent review of pesticide residues, 91% of the wheat sampled by the FDA contained pesticide residues! Wheat can be one of the most heavily treated grains, because it is stockpiled as a basic commodity and fumigated periodically to keep down pests. When it is milled, the outer coating—the bran included in whole wheat bread and cereals—is the portion which receives the most chemical treatment. The bran and germ portion of the wheat also retains the most residues. It has been suggested that some forms of so-called wheat allergy, which has been associated with learning problems and difficulty in concentrating, may actually be a neurotoxic reaction to the pesticide residues in the grain. These pesticides are, by definition, neurotoxins—that is how they affect the insects they are intended to destroy. Wheat is on this organic list because it is so heavily consumed by most people in this country and elsewhere throughout the world.

21. Eggs: These are typically produced in factory farms where the hens often live in unhygienic conditions. This may be one of the reasons that salmonella bacteria are found in eggs so frequently. More than 2 million eggs each year are contaminated, resulting in more than a half million cases of food poisoning. Factory farm eggs also may be lower in nutrients than organic ones, and they usually don't taste as good as farm fresh eggs from the free-ranging chickens that are not fed antibiotics. **Our best egg option is organic eggs, which are becoming more available in mainstream supermarkets.**

22. Seafood: Depending on where it is caught or harvested, seafood can be contaminated by polluted water. Since some chemicals persist in water (as well as in the soil), fish taken from pesticide-polluted water contain concentrations of the fat-soluble chemicals, including the estrogen-mimics. Rivers and lakes also contain other contaminants and heavy metals, including arsenic, cadmium, chromium, mercury, and lead. And sadly, more than 1,600 waterways are documented to be polluted with mercury. **If you are eating seafood regularly, be sure to consume a variety to avoid overexposure to specific chemicals or contaminants.**

23. Meat: This is reported by researchers to be one of the most contaminated products in our food supply. Like poultry, cattle and pigs no longer roam free, but are frequently raised under unsanitary feedlot conditions. Their health, productivity, and muscle mass are maintained by an array of drugs that include antibiotics, hormones, and steroids. They also receive antibacterials on their coats; additives and pesticides in their feed; and sedatives and other drugs for slaughter. If available, desirable, and affordable, choose less chemically-treated and cured meats and ideally, organically-raised meat, and be sure to store and cook it properly.

The next two entries may be a bit surprising, since those of you who have read *The Detox Diet* know that I don't support the regular intake of caffeine or alcohol. However, since I know many folks do partake regularly of these psychoactive substances, I feel that it is important to address them.

24. Coffee: The magic bean is often heavily treated with chemicals. Since people who drink coffee tend to do so regularly and often in quantity, there may be a significant risk of exposure to toxins. Coffee drinking is a questionable health habit, but if you are a regular coffee drinker, make that java organic and use good water.

HOW TO MINIMIZE PESTICIDES IN YOUR FOOD

- Limit use of out-of-season imported produce.

- Wash, soak, and peel conventionally grown fruits and vegetables.

- Limit your intake of red meats and factory-farmed poultry.

- Limit your intake of fish known to be caught from polluted waters.

- Replace some meat meals with complementary proteins such as corn, beans, whole grain rice, or soybeans and their products, such as tofu and tempeh.

- Buy some new bulk foods, such as beans, oats, and some time-honored grains that may be less treated, including millet, quinoa (keen-wah), barley, couscous, amaranth, and spelt.

- Try emphasizing fruits and vegetables that can be peeled or those that have been recently found to have low residues.

- Substitute one good fresh food for another. The Environmental Working Group has found that just twelve fruits and vegetables contain half the pesticide load in the average diet. The following chart includes a list of other fresh, nutritious foods you can substitute.

25. Wine: Grapes and wine may contain a variety of accumulated pesticides and other chemicals.* Likewise, many people who consume wine tend to be regular drinkers. Since it is thought that some of the adverse and hangover effects from wine drinking may be from the chemicals, try some organic wine, made from organically grown grapes, manufactured without chemicals or contaminated bottles and corks.

*Both grapes and wine—even organic wines—typically contain sulfites, so asthmatics and others sensitive to sulfites should consume only organic, sulfite-free wines if they choose to drink any alcohol.

ALTERNATIVES TO HEAVILY SPRAYED PRODUCE

Rank (1-most toxic)	Contaminated foods	Main nutrients	Alternative choices
1	Strawberries	Vitamin C	Blueberries, blackberries, oranges, grapefruit, cantaloupe (U.S.), kiwis, watermelon
2	Red and green bell peppers	Vitamin C	Green peas, broccoli, romaine lettuce
3	Spinach	Vitamins A & C	Broccoli, Brussels sprouts, romaine lettuce, asparagus
4	Cherries (U.S.)	Vitamin C	Oranges, blueberries, blackberries, grapefruit, cantaloupe, kiwis
5	Peaches	Vitamins A & C	Nectarines, cantaloupe, watermelon, tangerines, oranges, red or pink grapefruit
6	Cantaloupe (Mexican)	Vitamins A & C, Potassium	Buy U.S. cantaloupe in season (May to December) or watermelon
7	Celery	Sodium, Potassium	Carrots, romaine lettuce, broccoli, or radishes
8	Apples	Vitamin C	Pears (peeled or cooked), oranges, grapefruit, cantaloupe, kiwis, watermelon, nectarines, bananas, tangerines
9	Apricots	Vitamins A & C, Potassium	Nectarines, cantaloupe, watermelon, tangerines, oranges, red or pink grapefruit
10	Green beans	B Vitamins	Green peas, broccoli, cauliflower, Brussels sprouts, asparagus
11	Grapes (Chile)	Vitamin C	Buy U.S. grapes in season (May to Dec.)
12	Cucumbers	Minerals, some	Carrots, romaine lettuce, broccoli, radishes

10 THINGS YOU CAN DO TO HELP
THE ORGANIC MOVEMENT FLOURISH

1. Buy organic foods, especially those fruits and vegetables most heavily treated with chemicals.
2. Plant your own garden or organize and work in a community garden.
3. Shop at farmer's markets and get to know your local farmers. Be sure to ask the growers how their land and crops are treated. Even small farms may be heavy users of pesticides.
4. Find out if there's a buyer's co-op or a cooperative health food store in your area. (Community cooperative food stores typically give a discount in exchange for volunteer labor.)
5. Check alternative magazines and on the Internet for companies that ship or deliver seasonal organic produce through mail-order.
6. Eliminate pesticides and harsh chemicals from your home and garden.
7. Cut way back on meat and dairy because of the pesticide and chemicals that accumulate, particularly in the fats of these foods.
8. Read up on chemical concerns and their effects on humans and our planet. Some very fine books on this topic include: *Our Stolen Future, Toxic Deception, Generations at Risk, Designer Poisons,* and *Living Downstream. Organic Gardening Magazine*, a classic resource, is from Rodale Press, Inc., Emmaus, PA, 1-800-666-2206.
9. Get involved. Write letters to the FDA, EPA, and your local and national legislators. And remember, your dollar is your vote. Vote healthy.
10. Support organic farming and its advocates.

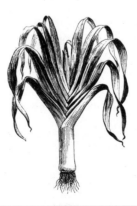

What to Do If You Can't Buy Organic

In some parts of the country, organic foods just aren't widely available. And for some of us, economics may preclude buying organic products. The next best option is a home or community garden. If you are limited to store-bought, nonorganic foods, thick-skinned fruits that we peel automatically, such as bananas, oranges, grapefruits, and avocados are good choices. You may want to consider peeling pears and other thin-skinned fruits, as well as waxed produce including apples, cucumbers, and peppers. (Waxing is used to hold in moisture.) Vegetables with skins or husks that must be removed, such as onions and corn, are also safer choices. Every diet should include cruciferous vegetables, although they are highly vulnerable to chemicals. So when choosing between cabbage and broccoli, for example, reach for the cabbage. The tough outer layers that you discard will reduce your exposure by protecting the tender inner leaves.

Resources

- The Organic Trade Association, Greenfield, MA, (413) 774-7511, <www.ota.com>

- California Certified Organic Farmers (CCOF), Santa Cruz, (408) 423-2263

- Committee for Sustainable Agriculture (CSA) sponsers an annual organic farming conference <www.csa.efc.org>

- Environmental Working Group (EWG), Washington, DC-based research group, (202) 667-6982, website: <www.ewg.org> Ask about *A Shopper's Guide to Pesticides in Produce*

- Food First, Oakland, CA, advocacy and health policy, publications (800) 274-7826. For information on the community food security movement, (510) 654-4400

- Mothers and Others: publications and advocacy—New York, (888) ECO-INFO, San Francisco, (415) 433-0850, <www.mothers.org/mothers>

- NCAMP, the National Coalition Against the Misuse of Pesticides, Washington, DC. To locate a consumer-owned marketing cooperative in your region, call (202) 543-5450

  Mail Order: Diamond Organics, (888) 674-2642, <www.diamondorganics.com>
  Walnut Acres, Penns Creek, PA, (800) 433-3998, <www.walnutacres.com>
  Seeds of Change, Santa Fe, MN, (800) 95-SEEDS

CHAPTER EIGHT

Safe Drinking Water

Just as we need for our food to be fresh, chemical-free, and nutritious, we want the water we drink to be clean and uncontaminated as well. Since water is second in importance only to the air we breathe in terms of sustaining our life, we don't want our drinking water laced with germs, pesticides, industrial chemicals, or heavy metals. Because water is the universal solvent, and most other substances present on Earth dissolve in it, pure water does not exist naturally on our planet. The Earth's natural waters vary in mineral content, just as our bodies vary in mineral status, and the water we choose to drink can affect that mineral balance.

Our bodies are at least 60% water. It is the primary component of all the body's fluids—lymph, urine, digestive juices, blood, sweat, and tears. Water is involved in almost every bodily function, including circulation, digestion, absorption, and the elimination of wastes. It is the medium in which all other nutrients are found and carries the mineral salts that help convey electrical currents in our body (electrolytes). The major minerals that make up these salts are sodium, potassium, calcium, magnesium, and chloride. Water requirements vary greatly from person to person based on the climate in which we live, our activity level, our body chemistry, and our diet.

Even though there are few studies on the specific benefits of water, it makes sense that clean water is essential to good health. Because water is so vital to our basic physiological needs, now is the time to support research and provide funds to keep our waters safe for human consumption.

My concern is that our governments will wait too long to correct our current water problems, much as modern medicine tends to focus on end-stage disease rather than preventive medicine. To heal and maintain the Earth's environment and safeguard our own physical health, we must support policies that ensure clean air, soil, and water.

WHAT'S WRONG WITH OUR WATER?

Clean drinking water has become an issue of serious concern. In all too many cases it has been shown that our drinking water is not totally safe. Research by the Environmental Working Group (EWG) in 1995 found that over 45 million Americans were supplied with tap water that failed to meet basic health standards. A similar study in 1994 had found that over 53 million Americans drank water that did not meet the standards set forth in the Safe Water Drinking Act. Federal and state records also show that the most common water impurities involve microbes, particularly bacteria such as E. coli, which affects the water supply of at least 35 million people. For another 5 million, levels of lead in the drinking water exceed the allowable standard (EWG). And numerous city water systems have been found to harbor microbes such as giardia and cryptosporidium, which can cause serious infections.

The Environmental Protection Agency provides monitoring and consumer information, although it labors under restrictive limitations on its advocacy role and as a catalyst for change. In the public sector, a number of conservation groups advocate

WATER CONTAMINATION CONCERNS

- **Chemicals from Industry**—Solvents, gasoline and other hydrocarbons, dioxin, PCBs, MTBE (a gasoline additive), asbestos, and plastics such as polyvinyl chloride
- **Agricultural Chemicals**—Fertilizers and chemical wastes in fertilizers, thousands of pesticides and herbicides (including carcinogens such as malathione, atrazine, alachlor and Aldicarb), plus DDT residues leaching from landfills and leaking storage tanks—gasoline, oil, and dumped chemicals
- **Radioactive Elements**—Uranium, radium, radon, and strontium
- **Metals**—Mining contamination, heavy metals from industry that include lead, mercury, arsenic, aluminum, cadmium, and chromium
- Contamination from water pipes that contain copper and lead or plastics
- **Chlorine and Fluoride**—and their byproducts such as THMs
- **Microbes in Reservoirs and other Water Sources**—From sewage and animal waste, bacteria, such as E. coli and listeria, viruses such as hepatitis A, and parasites, especially giardia and cryptosporidium
- **Soil Contamination**—Nitrates, sodium chloride, and selenium

on our behalf for clean water. These include the Environmental Working Group (EWG), Mothers and Others (M & O), Clean Water Action, and the National Resources Defense Council (NRDC).

Our primary water problems include contamination from microbes, heavy metals, industrial toxic wastes, and agricultural chemicals. Despite these potential threats to our health, the government and municipal water districts would still like us to believe that we should have no concerns about our drinking water.

Many physicians now believe that drinking tap water should be considered a risk factor for potential illness. Since 5 out of every 6 Americans use public water systems, this represents a major public health concern.

Technology can help us solve some of these problems. We have made significant progress in the development of systems to improve our drinking water, including improved chemical purification and water treatment systems, but we still have a way to go. I believe we must do better to insure our future.

TAP WATER

Most tap water comes from surface reservoirs formed from rivers, streams, and lakes, or from groundwater. Groundwater refers to the subterranean reservoirs that hold much of the Earth's water and supply nearly all rural drinking water and about half of city water supplies. The water from these sources goes through local treatment plants, many of which use a very old process involving settling tanks, filtration through sand and gravel, and then chemicals to clean the water so it is fit for human consumption.

Many minerals and chemicals are used for water "purification" (ridding the water of bacteria), including chlorine, alum or sodium aluminum salts, soda, ash, phosphates, and calcium hydroxide. Yet, this process may not eradicate all the many environmental pollutants that can contaminate our water supplies, including animal wastes, fertilizers and herbicides, insecticides, chemicals, toxic industrial wastes, and pollutants such as lead or radon. Chemicals and petroleum spills can also contaminate large amounts of water. Since much of this pollution affects groundwater deep in underground aquifers as well as surface waters, most municipal or artesian well drinking waters are at risk and deserve our attention. Areas of greatest concern include microbial and lead contamination.

It is quite clear that city tap water is now considered to be a processed, unnatural substance, containing potentially hazardous chemical additives as well as heavy metals and industrial pollutants. (No wonder bottled water has become a huge industry!) In most areas, city water is heavily chlorinated to kill germs, fluoridated to prevent tooth decay, and may contain added calcium hydroxide or other alkaline substances to change the acidity (pH) of the water so it doesn't corrode pipes.

For a variety of reasons, *I recommend that people not drink city or tap waters.* Public water treatment leaves much to be desired. Chlorine has become a panacea to treat and prevent contamination by microbes. Although this chemical treatment has helped rid our water of germs, it can also create additional problems because of the cancer-causing byproducts. *We must find better ways to clean public waters.* Ozone gas purification offers some potential, as it kills germs on contact, yet has no residual effect. It still requires some chlorine after it leaves the water plant, although far less than conventional purification using chlorine as the primary or sole treatment. At present, treating water in your home with a variety of systems just before drinking it is the safest way to assure that you're getting clean, chemical- and germ-free water.

We need to understand what role drinking tap water plays in our health. What is its subtle effect on biochemical processes in our body, and what is its relationship to symptoms of illness or chronic disease? The primary contaminates in our water include:

Microbes (Bacteria and Parasites)

At one time, we viewed water microbial contamination as a problem only in Third World countries. But microbial outbreaks in this decade have taught us that this problem is universal.

Germs—bacteria, viruses, and protozoa—are microscopic organisms that can enter drinking water from human sewage or animal waste. Parasitic amoebas and giardia, E. coli and other bacteria (from human and animal waste), and the hepatitis A virus (infectious hepatitis) infect close to a million people a year, frequently causing dysentary and killing hundreds, including children.

Two of the worst microbial offenders in our drinking water are *Giardia lamblia* and *Cryptosporidium parvum*, which can cause severe cramping and diarrhea, and may lead to dehydration or chronic gastrointestinal illness if undiagnosed. Several years ago in Milwaukee, over 400,000 were affected, more than 4,000 were hospitalized, and nearly 100 people died from cryptosporidium in the water (EPA).

Between 1971 and 1985, over 100,000 cases of disease in the United States were attributed to drinking water (Centers for Disease Control).

Recently, the CDC and the EPA advised anyone with a compromised immune system to consult their physician before drinking ordinary tap water! The American Water Works Association, a trade group representing water utilities, has advised all individuals with the HIV virus to boil tap water for 20 minutes before drinking it to prevent cryptosporidium and other microbe infections (EWG).

Lead

The primary source of lead in drinking water, which was used extensively in plumbing materials until the late 1980s, continues to be contaminated pipes (from the lead lining or soldering), still found in more than half the cities in the United States. Lead can damage an unborn fetus; in children, it can delay neurological and physical development; and in adults, it can cause high blood pressure, heart attacks, kidney damage, reproductive dysfunction, and strokes.

Government records indicate that lead is a common contaminant of water, affecting more than 5 million Americans. In addition to the corrosion of lead-lined or lead-soldered water pipes, lead gets into the drinking water from brass faucets. The possibility of contamination is of greatest concern to people living in homes more than 30 years old whose pipes may contain more lead, and for families with young children, since they are more sensitive to lead toxicity. **Testing for lead is relatively easy and inexpensive.** (See Resources at the end of this chapter.) **Reverse osmosis and solid carbon filters remove much of the lead, but distillation is the most efficient.** (See later discussion on Water Treatment Systems, page 137.)

Other Chemicals from Pipes

Plastic pipes leak more easily and may interact with industrial solvents, pesticides, or gasoline. Polyvinyl chloride (PVC), polybutylene (PB), and polyethylene (PE) are three common pipe plastics; the first two are mild carcinogens. Old asbestos cement (AC) pipes, of which some 200,000 miles were laid after World War II, can leak asbestos and may be associated with an increase in gastrointestinal cancer. Copper pipes may add excess copper to our bodies, and often have lead solder lines, which adds to lead contamination.

Industrial Waste

According to government records from the Toxics Release Inventory, more than 1 billion pounds of toxic chemical wastes were discharged directly into America's waters between 1990 and 1994 (EWG). As much as another estimated 450 million pounds were discharged indirectly into our waters from factories via sewage treatment plants.

Pesticides

A 1995 study in the Midwest, Louisiana, and Maryland found weed killers (herbicides) above the allowable level in more than thirteen cities (EWG). A 1997 study in the Midwest found that more than 100 communities, serving over 3 million people, had numerous (5 or more) toxic herbicides in their tap water. In one Ohio sample, researchers found 10 different pesticides and metabolites (EWG).

Nitrates (Byproducts of Agriculture)

As runoff from fertilizer, nitrates can heavily pollute our groundwater and drinking water in some areas. These waters may also have higher amounts of toxic pesticides and herbicides. In central California in 1998, water sources in farming areas were so badly contaminated with nitrates that the water was declared undrinkable. In 40 states across the country, nitrate contamination over the past decade was reported by the EPA for water sources that served more than 2 million people.

Nitrates can be converted to nitrites by our intestinal bacteria, creating highly carcinogenic nitrosamines in the body. Rural families, especially those with infants, and pregnant women, should test their water for nitrates. Nitrate-contaminated water can put infants at risk of "blue-baby" syndrome, a potentially fatal condition affecting the blood's ability to carry oxygen. **To clear nitrates from the water, both reverse osmosis filtration and distillation systems have been found to be effective.**

Fluoridated Water

Fluoridation of our water is a very controversial issue. The United States is currently the sole industrialized nation in the world still fluoridating much of its municipal water. The only positive thing that can be said for fluoride is that it does reduce dental cavities. However, this can also be accomplished with topical fluoride use in toothpaste, a better diet, and good oral hygiene. Risks from too much fluoride include bone problems, teeth mottling (called *fluorosis)*, and cancer. The element fluorine can also cause thyroid dysfunction, because it is related to iodine, which the thyroid depends upon for hormone production. ***Therefore, I am in not in favor of routinely drinking fluoridated or chlorinated water.*** Legal battles are being waged in a number of American cities between water authorities and consumers who wish to avoid fluoridated waters.

Chlorine

This and other additives used to treat water can react with organic chemicals to produce chlorinated hydrocarbons that may act as carcinogens. For example, chloramines (including chloroform and other trihalomethanes or THMs) are formed in water from chlorine and organic matter such as ammonia or decaying leaves. Chlorination of city reservoirs is routine in much of the United States.

In March 1998, the medical journal, *Epidemiology*, reported two studies about the risks of chlorinated water that shocked even the most conservative politicians. As reviewed in the journal *Alternative Medicine* in July 1998, these studies found that miscarriage rates were nearly double in women who drank chlorinated water contaminated with over 75 parts per million (ppm) of THMS (which is not uncommon in tap waters) over those who did not drink tap water. There were even higher miscarriage rates when the THMs went up near 150 ppm.

Several other studies have shown an increased incidence of cancer, especially of the gastrointestinal tract and rectum, in people who drank chlorinated water. THMs may be associated with the 10,000 or more gastrointestinal and bladder cancers each year in the U.S. and are linked to pancreatic cancer as well. These chemicals may also cause serious birth defects (M&O). And this is probably just the tip of the iceberg. The EPA has determined that essentially all of our chlorinated water supplies contain these toxic THMs. Chloroform, for example, a common THM chemical, is often found in city waters. Since nearly 80% of our country drinks chlorinated water, this is an important issue for our national health.

Another chlorination issue relating to THMs involves the chemical gases that we inhale when we take hot showers. We can absorb even higher amounts of THMs from showers than from drinking water! **There are special dechlorinating filters that can be attached to shower heads to remedy this potential risk. The KDF (Kinetic-Degradation-Fluxion) filter was specifically designed for this purpose.**

Radon

This is a radioactive gas byproduct of uranium and is found in the Earth's crust. High radon gas levels are associated with an increased risk of lung cancer. This carcinogenic element can be present in household tap water but is more likely to be found in the northeastern United States, North Carolina, and Arizona. Water that comes from wells and groundwater has a higher incidence of radon contamination. Municipal waters that come from lakes, rivers, and reservoirs are usually low in radon. When present in the water, radon can be released into the air during showering, laundering, and dish washing. Radon in the air at home can be tested with several new low-cost devices on the market. If present in the water in high amounts, **radon can be removed with carbon filtration, but this must be attached to the entire home water system. Shower devices are also available to remove some chemicals, chlorine, and radon.**

WATER TESTING

Water is such an important issue that you would think there would be continued testing, frequent studies, and copious information available to us. At the very least, water companies should guarantee their water and check it regularly for contaminants. They should supply us with their testing results on request, especially if we are using their product as our main source of drinking water. **Information on the water quality in your area can be obtained from the municipal water districts and from the web site of the Environmental Working Group (www.ewg.org) or from the online "Chemical Scorecard" from the Environmental Defense Fund (www.scorecard.org).**

If you live in a dense city or industrial area, you should be wary of your tap water. If your water has an odd or unpleasant taste or odor or stains your tub or sink, *have it checked.* It is fairly inexpensive to have the bacteria count of your water verified. Analyzing water for chemicals can be more difficult and costly. There are very few companies that perform this service and it can cost hundreds of dollars to check for more toxic chemical contaminants, such as the organic halides, trihalomethanes (THMs), vinyl chloride (VC), trichloroethylene (TCE), ethylene dibromide (EDB), and dibromo-chloropropane (DBCP). There are many others.

It may be worthwhile to analyze questionable water for toxic chemicals and metals, as well as to analyze its mineral content, hardness, and pH. (See Resources at the end of the chapter for a list of companies that test water.)

WATER CONTAMINATION AND TREATMENT CHOICES

Toxin	US Population Affected (94-95)	Who Is Potentially Affected?	Water Treatment Choices
Bacteria	25 million	Anyone	Distillation, ozone, UV light, and ultrafiltration*
Chemicals, Industrial	1 million	Anyone	Distillation, carbon filtration, and reverse osmosis (RO)
Chlorine and potential THMs	at least 80 to 120 million	More than half of municipal systems	Most methods; RO only with carbon
Fluoride	Approximately 128 million	In about 62% of the water systems	Distillation best, RO is also good
Lead and other heavy metals	5 million	Old houses, old water systems, industrial areas	Distillation best, RO good, Carbon is fair
Nitrates	500,000	Agricultural areas	Distillation and RO
Parasites	giardia (2 million) cryptosporidum (estimated 5-6 mil.)	Anyone	Distillation surest, Carbon† or RO† may work 1 micron filter or smaller
Pesticides	At least 1 million	Agricultural areas	RO, carbon & distillation
Radioactivity, radon, and other elements	about 300,000 88 water systems	Anyone linked to certain water systems	Solid carbon and Distillation
Trihalomethanes (THMs)	At least 600,000	In chlorinated water	Solid carbon, or RO & distillation w/ carbon
Volatile Organic Compounds	600,000	Anyone, particularly consumers of groundwater	Distillation with carbon prefilter, RO w/ carbon may be the best petroleum byproducts

*designed for bacterial removal.
†some are certified by the National Sanitation Foundation (NSF).
Source: Earth Working Group Website; information from federal and state records from July 1994 through June 1995. These are just the reported figures in government records.

CHOOSING YOUR DRINKING WATER

I have urged people for many years to use purified and filtered drinking water and to avoid the faucet. The word "purifier" is a specific state and federal legal term for any system that actually destroys bacteria. A filter may do a good job of clearing bacteria, however, it cannot be called a purifier because bacteria remain in the system and can be released back into the water. Distillation is a purifying process, as bacteria are destroyed with boiling.

Lately there have even been questions in the media regarding the purity of bottled waters and the effectiveness of filters. Not surprisingly, scientific research and the marketing information of companies selling water or filters often differ. The government can only protect the consumer from gross misrepresentation and not subtle interpretation of "facts."

Providing safe and tasty drinking water has become a burgeoning industry, largely due to widespread concerns over tap water. In every grocery store and supermarket, we now find domestic and international spring waters, designer waters, flavored waters, juice waters, and more. At least 1 in 6 Americans uses bottled water as their main drinking source. And in a 1997 survey by the Water Quality Association, 1 in 3 adults (32%) surveyed reported using some kind of water treatment device, up from 27% in 1995. So, which is safer—bottled or home treated water? And which water treatment system or bottled water should you choose?

Bottled Waters

Bottled water is more likely to have fewer toxic chemicals than tap water, but it too can come from contaminated groundwater. Sometimes, it is merely filtered city tap water. Many waters are bottled from artesian wells and natural underground springs from around the world. (An artesian well is reached by drilling through impenetrable strata providing water that then naturally rises to the Earth's surface.) Let's first consider the various sources of bottled water.

Well Water

Well water comes primarily from groundwater supplies and can vary greatly in its mineral content; it also is vulnerable to whatever chemicals seep into the Earth. Some well waters are very low in minerals while others contain a variety of beneficial nutrients such as iron, zinc, selenium, magnesium, or calcium, all of which could affect our body's mineral levels. More than 23 million Americans use groundwaters as their primary drinking water source.

Unfortunately, well water is not necessarily safe, either. The groundwater source from which it comes may also contain toxic metals or agricultural and industrial chemical pollutants such as pesticides, herbicides, radon, asbestos, or hydrocarbons (gasoline byproducts). In recent years, many thousands of wells have been closed in over half of the states throughout the country because of contamination, and those are only the ones that have been discovered; there may be many more. Living in the country does not assure that you are isolated from chemicals, especially if you live in an agricultural area. Even if you have been using a particular well for a number of years, it is now necessary to check the water for chemicals, microbes, and minerals; your life could depend on it. Then, with a clean bill of health and periodic testing, you can feel free to use this water that is readily available to you and your family.

Spring Water

This is the "natural" water found in surface or underground springs. Some companies retrieve and bottle this water. This water may be filtered or disinfected with chlorine, and if so, it is no longer spring water, but "drinking water." The unchlorinated spring waters typically taste very different from tap water and, to me, are a refreshing drink. The mineral content depends upon the region from which the water is taken and whether it is surface or underground water (surface spring water is relatively low in minerals). Naturally found minerals in spring waters are thought to support mineral levels and mineral metabolism in the body; in fact, they may be closer to "colloidal" minerals which are more bioavailable in that they are bound to organic materials, such as plant cells and tissues. (However, there is still some controversy over this idea in that much of these ionized minerals bound with the water are not usable, and there may not be enough to really make any difference.) For example, the lakes, streams, and spring water from the southeastern and northwestern regions of our country are relatively low in minerals, and this "soft" water may increase the incidence of cardiovascular disease. The Midwest, by contrast, has high-mineral underground waters, and the farming community who drink this mineral-rich unchlorinated water through their wells have a lower rate of cardiovascular disease. Of course, there may be other lifestyle factors that may contribute to this finding.

Just as groundwater can be polluted, spring water can also be contaminated. **It is a good idea to request summaries of tests from the company selling the spring water, particularly if you are planning to use their water as your primary source.** (Beginning in 1998, European waters will be held to a different (less strict) standard for bottled water than American waters.) Ideally, they have independent lab reports, which are performed regularly. You may also want to ask if the water is bottled at the source or transported and then treated and bottled. Water bottled at the source is preferable. Although spring waters can be costly, many people enjoy them.

Mineral Water

Essentially, most waters are mineral waters—that is, they contain minerals. In California, the standard for bottled mineral water is more than 500 ppm (parts per million) of dissolved minerals. Underground bubbly water, called "natural sparkling water," usually contains lots of minerals, as well as carbon dioxide (CO_2). Many companies bottling this "mineral" water must inject CO_2 back into the water, since it is easily lost between the surface and the bottle.

Carbonated Water

"Seltzer" identifies any water that is carbonated with carbon dioxide; it is often made from filtered tap water. Club soda is essentially the same, though it frequently has more minerals added. All of these types of waters can also be polluted, although any bottled carbonated water should be free of microorganisms because they cannot easily live in the presence of higher levels of carbon dioxide. I do not recommend drinking large amounts of carbonated waters because the carbon dioxide can affect the body's acid-alkaline balance.

Packaging Issues

Water containers offer another potential biochemical risk. Polyethylene, a soft plastic commonly used for many water containers, can contaminate water, but the level of this toxicity is relatively low. However, if the water has sat in the container for a long time, then the plastic contaminants may be at a higher level. Plastics can also absorb small amounts of chemicals, from gasoline to dish detergents and cleaning fluids, which could have some ill effects with regular exposure.

The 5-gallon plastic jugs used to deliver water are made of polycarbonate (a harder and thicker plastic than polyethylene). Bisphenol-A, a plastic byproduct known to disrupt hormones just as pesticides do, can be leached from this type of plastic (M&O). Methylene chloride, another toxic chemical, is used as a binder in plastic and can contaminate the water also. These plastic byproducts are released in greatest amounts when the plastic is exposed to high temperatures or caustic cleaners, according to 1993 research from Stanford University.

HOME WATER TREATMENT SYSTEMS

In the long run, home water filters are the least expensive and safest way to obtain good drinking water. Most are reasonably priced and will remove many of the harmful chemicals in your tap water. However, be sure to obtain information about a filter before you buy it, such as cost, longevity, percentage removal, filter changes, recyclability, etc. Research in 1998 found that some of the most popular water filters on the market actually *increased* the levels of lead in the water, due to lead solder within the faucets or design flaws (such as the "unloading" phenomenon, meaning a system first collects and then dumps a particular material). This "unloading" may be a concern with microbes, as some filters may harbor bacteria and then release them into the water. Therefore, it is important that filters be kept clean and changed regularly. (See Resources)

Filtration and purification involve the removal of extraneous matter from water, be it chemicals, metals, or bacteria. Legally, anything called a "purifier" must remove (actually destroy) 99.75% of incoming bacteria. Most filters cannot be termed purifiers. Americans are purchasing about 2 million home water treatment systems yearly, and there are a great many models from which to choose.

Water can be filtered using a number of methods: carbon block filters, reverse osmosis, distillers, and water ionizers that create alkalinized water. Filtering systems come in models made for the countertop, to fit directly on the faucet or under the sink, and in a portable pitcher/carafe style. The two main types of carbon filters are **granulated carbon** and **solid carbon block** filters. Solid carbon block filtration is a good basic system that will remove most chemicals. Avoid granulated carbon filters, although they are better than nothing. **Reverse osmosis filters** are also a good choice; however, these systems usually have three different filters and tend to be more expensive. Reverse osmosis also needs good water pressure and wastes water, plus their performance can vary depending upon the water source. **Distilled water may be the most reliable source for clean drinking water,** although the distillation process does take an effort to make daily water. It is obvious that we have more to learn. So be sure to educate yourself about water treatment before purchasing a home unit.

Activated Carbon (AC)

Carbon is the most widely used type of filter. The carbon, used for centuries as a filtering substance, is treated to provide a large surface area with which to attach (adsorb) contaminants. Most carbon units filter the water mechanically and biomagnetically (ionically) and eliminate the unpleasant appearance, odor, and taste by removing bacteria, parasites, chlorine, and particulate matter. Carbon is best at removing organic chemicals and chlorine. The size of the filter determines the particles it will separate. Carbon filters will remove any particles or organisms from 0.2 to 0.5 microns (size of filter pores), which is most bacteria and parasites, although not viruses. However, bacteria may stay in the system and be reintroduced into the drinking water, so AC cannot be deemed a purifier and is not acceptable for bacteria removal. Carbon is excellent at electrically binding larger molecules, chemicals, and larger microorganisms; however, it does not remove inorganic minerals such as the fluoride typically found in municipal waters.

The **granulated carbon filter** has air spaces between the carbon particles, which can hold bacteria and allow it to multiply within these air spaces. Silver is used in some granulated filters to assist in killing the bacteria. These "silver-impregnated" filters do help reduce the bacterial growth within the filter, but there are concerns about ineffectiveness and about silver toxicity, and this bacteria-inhibiting effect may be short term. **Although granulated carbon filters are economical, their use is short-lived, and their safety is definitely questionable; I do not recommend them. However, they do have a place as a component in more complete water treatment systems.**

The dense **solid carbon block filter** alleviates most of the concern with microorganism contamination. The filtering surface area of this denser carbon bed can clean much more water, but inactive microbes can collect within the filter and be released back into the water. **Therefore, if the filter is not used for a day or longer, let the water run through it for 20 to 30 seconds to be safe before drinking.** Research has demonstrated that these units also clear more chemicals, organic pollutants, radon, and asbestos than the looser, granulated carbon filters. The solid carbon block removes chemicals, giardia and crypto cysts, and chlorine, but not fluoride. Certain carbon block filters are enhanced with resins to combat specific problems, such as fluoride, water hardness, iron, lead, and other heavy metals. Solid carbon filters are usually more expensive than the granulated type.

Carbon filters are rated by the volume of water treated, since they can hold only a limited amount of sediment. Most carbon filters clean from 400 to 1,000 gallons of water, although each unit will vary depending on the amount of organic material in the incoming water. **It is essential to change the filter periodically, because it can collect and then release bacteria and sediment back into the water.** This can also happen with release of THMs. **Hot water should not be run through carbon filters because it can cause contaminant release.** It is suggested that filters be changed every six months. If the filter is getting too full, the water flow slows. The filter cartridge should probably be changed at about 75% of its maximum capacity for best results. Figure your average daily usage and mark the time for replacement on your calendar. Activated carbon filters, although more expensive than tap water, are usually less expensive (about 5 cents a gallon) than distillers or units that use reverse osmosis.

Kinetic-Degradation-Fluxion (KDF)

This is a relatively new type of metallic synthetic filter, originally designed to remove chlorine from shower water. It actually works better with hot water, while most carbon blocks work best with cold water. In addition to chlorine, the KDF also removes some of the other contaminants including lead and other metals. The concern is that KDFs do not remove the THMs from the shower water, which may be worse for us than chlorine. They also have a problem with clumping of particulate material, so if you have excess particulates in your water, choose another system. KDF seems to work best for shower dechlorinators. When used for drinking water, this method may result in a bitter taste.

Reverse Osmosis (RO)

Thought by many to be the best way to filter water, this is a multistage system in which tap water flows through special membranes containing microporous holes the size of the water molecule. These pores allow water molecules to pass through while rejecting the larger inorganic and organic materials. Reverse osmosis is a type of filtration that can clear much of the excess lead from the water. In fact, RO tends to remove almost all unwanted particles, including most chemicals as well as chlorine, and is one of the few water filtration methods that removes at least a portion of the fluoride. There is some concern with bacterial overgrowth, especially if the system is used infrequently or if filters are not changed periodically.

Reverse osmosis units usually have three or four filtering mechanisms. The first is a sedimentation filter, which traps particles. The second is either the RO membrane or a carbon filter (for chlorine), and the last is another one or two carbon filters, which remove most of the organic contaminants (and chlorine) that may have passed through the RO membrane, which improves the overall taste and odor. With this system, virtually 100% of the organic material is removed, along with almost all the minerals. **Reverse osmosis filters need to be cleaned or replaced every six months to a year, based on usage.** This adds to the initial costs, which tend to be higher than other types of filtration systems, at least $400 to $500 for a good unit. (The RO unit can last several years based on the quality of the feed water.)

Reverse osmosis units range from small home units to those of industrial size. Home units can make from 3 to 10 gallons of water a day. They are also energy efficient, as they require only tap water pressure. However, they are not water efficient as they require 3 to 5 gallons of water for each gallon made. The cost of RO drinking water is 30 to 40 cents per gallon based on needs of 3 to 5 gallons day, and this includes water waste and filter changes, about once yearly.

Another concern with RO units is that they remove almost all the minerals in water, including the good ones. Many authorities consider such minerals to be an important and healthful component in our water. They are concerned that drinking water, devoid of minerals, may negatively affect our body's mineral balance and electrolyte activity. This issue needs to be better researched, particularly if RO home water filtration is your primary source of drinking water. Nonetheless, the current consensus is that RO water is not a problem if you eat a balanced diet and have adequate mineral intake. This can be assessed by your doctor who may recommend that you take an appropriate mineral supplement.

Distillation

Distillation is a reliable process for filtration *and* purification. The distillation process involves vaporizing water (turning it into steam) in one chamber and then condensing it once again into liquid in a separate chamber. This removes the minerals, chemicals, and microbes from the water. Distilled water should be very close to pure H_2O. However, there is some concern that certain volatile organic chemicals will vaporize and recondense into the second chamber's water; therefore, distillation should be preceded by solid carbon filtration. Home distillers can be fairly expensive, although prices have become more competitive in recent years. Distillation requires electrical energy to process a few gallons, and it takes significant time, usually several hours per gallon, for the water to be distilled, thus limiting the amount available for use. It will, however, do a complete and consistent job no matter what type of water is presented.

There is a controversy I have expressed in previous books that distilled water may adversely affect mineral activity in the body and have a different bioelectrical effect. Observation and reports from clinicians who assess this bioelectrical phenomenon indicate that distilled water may not always be beneficial to health. The regular consumption of distilled water may cause mineral deficiencies, and aggravate anyone who is already depleted. Fasting for long periods exclusively on distilled water is not recommended because of the potential mineral depletion. Another school of thought suggests that distilled water may actually be healthier because the water molecules form a hexagonal configuration, which appears to be ideal for healthy body function and apparently hydrates cells and tissues better. Distilled water may be suggested during detoxification diets because it can be more effective for this process, having a stronger tendency to draw toxins out of the body. Also, when making herbal teas, distilled water may help bring out the most in the medicinal properties of the herbs.

Some nutritional advocates (mostly "old school" practitioners) recommend drinking demineralized water because they believe that the inorganic minerals contained naturally in mineral waters are not usable by the human body, and may even cause health problems. Research indicates that this is simply not true. Inorganic minerals and mineral salts can still be partially dealt with by our digestive tracts, and then assimilated and used by the body. The mineral levels in water, however, aren't nearly sufficient to satisfy the body's needs. Cooking foods in demineralized water will pull more minerals from the food, whereas using water containing natural minerals will lessen this loss and possibly even improve food values. Furthermore, the dissolved solids such as the trace minerals selenium, zinc, or silica, found in natural waters are associated with lower cancer rates in the people who consume them. Many of the cultures whose people live long healthy lives are located in regions with mineral-rich mountain water. Overall, I believe that the naturally occurring earth minerals contained in pure waters are beneficial to our health.

Ionized "Microwater"

The Japanese have developed a water system that polarizes water into alkaline and acid components through ionization, or "electrolysis." This ancient biochemical process is now technically adapted to provide filtered alkaline drinking water, which helps to balance the acidic condition that naturopathic practitioners believe is correlated with chronic degenerative disease. By alkalinizing the body with water and a diet higher in fruits and vegetables, it is thought to move the body toward healing. The ionized water is also reduced rather than oxidized, which means it can receive electrons, such as those found in damaging free radicals, much like helpful nutritional antioxidants do. Also, the acidic waters that are left from this ionization process can be used for cleaning and disinfecting, scrubbing away molds, and other purposes.

Ozonated Water

Ozone has been used as a disinfectant for water. Because it generates free radicals, it can kill bacteria. It is often used in place of chlorine in pools and spas. **However, drinking water with ozone in it, or other free radical generators, such as hydrogen peroxide, can have toxic effects and is not recommended.**

WATER SAFETY FOR TRAVELING AND CAMPING

When traveling or camping in more remote areas of this country, we need to take measures to make the water safe from microorganisms. Untreated water may harbor bacteria, parasites, or viruses. Our mountain rivers, streams, and lakes may contain parasites such as giardia, cryptosporidium, and amoebas, as well as E. coli and other bacteria. We can, in turn, become infected either by drinking or swimming in the water. Contracting hepatitis from contaminated water is another concern.

We have a few options concerning drinking water when we travel. We can carry our own water, although this is limited to short trips or when camping with a vehicle. We can also avoid drinking water altogether as some do, for example, when traveling to Mexico or South America. Drinking bottled carbonated beverages such as sparkling waters, sodas, and beer usually keeps us safe from germs, as they cannot exist in the high carbon dioxide levels. But contaminated water used to wash food or to make ice cubes can cause serious illness.

There are three primary ways to clean water to make it safer—heat, chemicals, and filtration. At sea level, boiling water for 1 minute will kill bacteria and parasites; boiling for 10 minutes will destroy viruses. To be on the safe side then, boil the water 10 minutes. For every 1,000 feet of elevation, add 1 minute to the boiling time to clean the water of possible germs. So at an altitude of 10,000 feet, water must be boiled for about 20 minutes.

Chemical treatment may be the simplest and the least expensive method for cleaning water while traveling, yet it has drawbacks. Chemically treated water does not taste very good, and some people might have side effects or reactions. Both chlorine and iodine have been used effectively to make water safe for drinking. Halazone tablets release chlorine into the water. Five tablets per quart will effectively kill almost all microorganisms, but the taste is not very exciting. In my opinion, iodine is preferable. Use 10 drops per quart of the 2% solution and let it sit for 30 minutes to kill the germs. Globaline is a crystalline iodine. One tablet can be added to 1 quart of water and will work in 10 minutes. Overall, I believe that chemical treatment is a last resort for water purification. But it is important to use this method while camping or when traveling if other water purification resources are impractical or unavailable.

Our goal at home or when traveling is to have germ-free water without chemicals or chlorine.

There are also water filters designed for travel and camping. These are small units that have pumps so that lake or river water can be used. Because about 2 million people a year contract giardia, many by drinking from crystal clear mountain streams, **wilderness packers need to carry some type of water purification.** Given the difficulty of boiling water at higher altitudes and the less optimal taste of chemically purified water, filtration is the best way to go for backpacking, especially if large amounts of water are needed.

Most hand filters are granulated carbon, often with silver added. Although these are not ideal for home use, they are the simplest for travel. They will take out some chemicals, but our biggest concern is microorganisms. The pore size of the filter is the crucial factor in determining what germs will be removed. Check the product information carefully.

MICROBES & MICRONS TABLE	
Organism	**Size in microns**
Giardia lamblia	10-20
Amoebas	10-50
Cryptosporidium	2-5
Campylobacter bacteria	.2-.3
CMV and Herpes virus	.15-.2
Retro virus (AIDS)	.1-.12
Hepatitis viruses	.025-.04

The pore size of available portable filters ranges from 0.2 to 2.0 microns. They all will remove parasites, some will remove bacteria, but most will not take out viruses. Since viruses are less likely to survive in water, they are really a lesser concern. (The Katadyn unit, claiming a pore size of .2 microns, may actually remove some viruses.) Most of the available travel filters can clean about 1 to 2 pints per minute. **If the water is dirty or turbid, use a prefilter such as a coffee filter or clean cotton bandanna, for example, and pour the water through one of these before pumping. This prefiltering also extends the life of the carbon filter.**

HOW MUCH WATER SHOULD WE DRINK?

Drinking the right amount of water is also crucial to our health. All the beverages we drink—teas, coffee, sodas, beer, juices, etc.—are basically water that contains other ingredients for flavor or nutrition. But I believe that drinking good water is still the best way to obtain our fluid requirements.

The amount of water we need is determined by a number of factors—our activity level, which influences the amount of fluid we lose through perspiration; our physical size; the climate in which we live (higher temperatures increase our fluid losses); and our diet. An inactive, small person living in a cool climate needs less water than a larger person who is an athlete training in the desert. It's also important to remember that a diet high in fruits and vegetables provides more fluids than a diet high in fat, meats, and dairy products. Special circumstances in which

SAFE WATER TIPS

1. Avoid drinking tap water, including chlorinated and fluoridated waters, as your main drinking source.
2. Drink either bottled water or filtered water, depending on your family's needs and budget.
3. Consider having your regular drinking water professionally assessed.
4. If you're puzzled about which water system to use, choose the reverse osmosis with a post-carbon filter.
5. If you shower regularly with chlorinated water, invest in a dechlorinator and filter attachment for the shower.
6. When traveling, be extra careful about contaminated water. Boiling it for 15 to 20 minutes will get rid of most germs. Allowing water to sit in the open air can release the chlorine gas and some chemicals. Or you can use iodine tablets or an appropriate travel filtration system.
7. If you must drink water from older pipes, avoid the first morning's water. Let it run for a minute or two first to avoid the potential copper and lead that might have been released into the water that sat overnight in the pipes.
8. Avoid using tap water in baby formulas and young children's foods. Never use hot tapwater, which can contain even more lead.
9. Read up on drinking water issues in sources such as *Save Our Planet* by Diane MacEachern and *Healthy Water for a Longer Life* by Martin Fox.

increased amounts of water may be needed include fever, diarrhea, kidney disease, or any situation where excessive fluid losses occur.

We lose water daily through our skin, bladder, bowels, and even our lungs (as water vapor in the air). About half of our water losses can be replaced with the water content in our food. The remaining half requires specific fluid intake, primarily from drinking good water. Caffeinated beverages, such as coffee, tea, cocoa, and colas, and alcoholic beverages do not count as the same volume of water because they act as diuretics in the body, increasing fluid losses from the kidneys.

In addition to a healthy diet containing fresh fruits and vegetables, I recommend that the average person consume at least 6 to 8 cups of water daily. I also suggest a physically active lifestyle with daily exercise. Water is best consumed at several intervals throughout the day—one or two glasses upon awakening and also about an hour before each meal. Water should not be drunk with or just after meals, as it can dilute digestive juices and reduce food digestion and nutrient assimilation. Some people, as I do, like to drink a glass or two in the evening to help flush out their systems overnight, even though this may result in getting up during the night to urinate. It is important to drink sufficient water to avoid problems such as constipation and dry skin. Drinking enough contaminant-free water is probably one of the most significant contributions we can make to our nutritional health as it helps with detoxification and circulation of nutrients to our cells and tissues.

Because good drinking water is so essential to good health, we must educate ourselves about the water we consume and what it contains. If there is any question about the water you drink, have it checked for bacteria count, mineral content, and the presence of chemical pollutants; then find a treatment system that makes your water safe to drink, or buy bottled water. If you can afford it, consider purchasing a home water filter system or having bottled water delivered. If economics precludes these options, develop a routine for boiling your water each day to protect your health.

Resources

Tap water quality in your area: *EPA's Safe Drinking Water Hotline* (800) (426-4791) Operators can provide you with a source for locating certified testing facilities in your state or help you interpret local public water test results.

Tap water research: The Environmental Working Group's web site provides six studies by EWG on drinking water issues, and a review of the water safety violations that have occurred in most states over the past decade, listed by county, at <www.ewg.org>.

Tap water quality: Specific information on water safety can also be obtained from Environmental Defense Fund <www.scorecard.org> Another supportive organization is Clean Water Action, Washington, DC (202) 895-0420.

Bottled water quality: The International Bottled Water Association (IBEW) in Virginia (1-703-683-5213 or 1-800-928-3711)—Bottlers of water need to meet certain standards to be part of the IBEW, and they may be able to provide you with a list of members or give you information about a particular water.

Bottled water is regulated by the FDA, which can provide information at (800) 332-4010 or (800) 532-4440.

Water filtration information is available from the following:

National Sanitation Foundation: (NSF) (800) 673-8010 or (313) 769-8010

Water Quality Association: (WQA) (800) 749-0234 or (888) 505-0160

Sources for bottled water and filtration systems: Check the Yellow Pages, search the Internet for <water filters>, or try one of the mail order companies that sell natural products, such as Inner Balance at (800) 482-3608 or Harmony (800) 456-1139. Also, many local stores sell water filtration systems, and in some cities, there are entire stores devoted to water.

More information on water filters: A thorough article on water filtration systems was published in *Consumer Reports*, July 1997.

More information on public water systems: The American Water Works Association serves water systems with technical information. Their web site address <www.awwa.org>

Water Testing Resources

If you live in a city, municipal water systems will often test water for free.

If you live in a more rural area and have well water, the Department of Public Health will test your water for bacteria and metals at no cost.

The following labs are nationally accredited and will test water from anywhere for a fee.

CSL Water Treatment, Inc., Warren, NJ (908) 647-1400

National Testing Laboratory, OH (800) 458-3330

Suburban Water Testing, Temple, PA (800) 433-6595

Spectrum Laboratories, St. Paul, MN (800) 633-0101 or (612) 633-0101

Water Treatment Systems are available through local stores. Some cities actually have stores that sell all the systems and paraphernalia for water. Several companies sell water treatment systems via mail order or offer consultants to help you choose your best options.

Aqua Technology, San Jose, CA (800) 478-7342

The Water Store, Greenbrae, CA (800) 776-7654

Real Goods, Hopland, CA (800) 749-0252

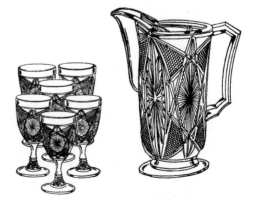

CHAPTER NINE

Staying Healthy in the Kitchen

◆

FOOD PREPARATION & HYGIENE

Most of us spend a significant part of our lives shopping for food, preparing meals, and consuming the byproducts of our efforts. For many of us, mealtime is an important ritual, while food preparation and cleanup are usually considered mundane and tedious tasks. Yet, being lax in these important chores can pose very serious risks to our health. As you read this chapter, I hope you will be encouraged to regard your work in the kitchen as a meaningful contribution to your family's good health. Realizing this, I think you will carry out these daily chores with a higher sense of purpose and pride.

A NEW OUTLOOK IN FOOD PREPARATION

- *The mindfulness of cooking*: Food preparation and hygiene are a reflection of our awareness and attentiveness to other aspects of our lives.
- *The elegance of cleanliness*: Even a simple meal can be quite beautiful if it is composed of wholesome ingredients and attractively arranged. However, it is difficult to create elegance when the kitchen or dining areas are cluttered or unclean.
- *The rituals of handling food*: There are certain rituals associated with kitchen hygiene and food preparation that have kept people from harm since time remembered.
- *Creating order in our lives*: The more organized we are, the less likely we will be to have contamination. An orderly kitchen allows greater efficiency in all aspects of cooking and cleanup.

Our Changing Microbial World

When it comes to proper hygiene in the kitchen, we are generally aware of the basics, such as keeping countertops, cupboards, and appliances clean; cooking certain foods to make them safe for consumption; refrigerating particular food items so that they won't spoil; and washing our hands before handling food. These sensible habits are usually second nature to anyone who spends any time preparing food and cleaning up after meals.

What may not be so obvious to most of us is a threat that looms large even in today's modern kitchen: greater exposure to potentially harmful microbes. There are now antibiotic-resistant microorganisms, emerging pathogens (such as E. coli 0157:H7), and old invaders making a comeback. Familiar pathogens are contaminating foods previously thought to be safe, such as orange juice and alfalfa sprouts. So it is essential that we adapt our kitchen habits to this changing microbial world to which we're exposed.

The best way to cope with germ problems is to prevent them. We want to avoid infections with E. coli and other invisible, microscopic bacteria, molds, and viruses by washing and cooking them away. Otherwise, if they get into the body, they can cause infection and require treatment.

Why are microbes an increasing health hazard? We now live in a global society where world travel and trade are commonplace. Millions of people travel internationally each year and rapid transport means that infections are spread more rapidly. And a quarter of our food supply comes from overseas and outside our borders. In fact, depending on the season, up to 70% of the fruits and vegetables consumed in the U.S. come from Mexico and South America. When we import food, we import an entire microbial population.

We also live in an overpopulated society—90% of us reside and/or work in crowded cities. Germs can spread quickly in densely populated areas. And our food is processed on a massive scale as well, in batches of millions of pounds, that are often shipped thousands of miles. Because of consumer demand and the global food market, ingredients from many countries may be combined in a single dish, which makes any contamination difficult to track. Furthermore, microbes are highly adaptable and respond to these opportunities. Simple transgressions in the kitchen can make the food unsafe. And because some produce and products have a short shelflife, it may be gone before an outbreak is recognized (a concern of the CDC).

So microbe contamination in our food supply is an area of growing concern. There have been an increasing number of cases which have been more difficult to treat because some organisms have become resistant to our common antibiotics and require stronger, more expensive, and more toxic drug therapies.

From 1973 to 1987, tainted produce accounted for just 2% of foodborne illness. But from 1988 through 1991, it caused 5% of the outbreaks. Recent contaminations indicate that these problems are on the rise and have been linked to apple juice and cider, strawberries and raspberries, lettuce and tomatoes, ground beef and other beef products. The safety of our food supply has become a major public health problem.

WHO'S IN CHARGE?

The government has responded to the rising incidence of illness and fatalities with legislation and funding to increase the authority of the agencies that monitor our food. The Food and Drug Administration (FDA) regulates some canned goods, imported produce, pasteurized milk, many seafoods, and meals on aircraft and trains. The U.S. Department of Agriculture regulates meat, poultry, and pasteurized eggs, and investigates animal and plant diseases. The CDC assesses risk for public health hazards, conducts national surveillance, and launches epidemic response in support of state health departments.

But they can only do so much. Most food processing plants are inspected once every 10 years. One or two of every 100 shipments of imported food are tested in a lab. So we are best protected if we do our part as well, by using good hygiene and careful food handling as a protection against illness.

Food Contamination and Food Poisoning

Although only about 100,000 cases of food poisoning are reported to the CDC each year, many more cases actually occur. Their estimate is that the occurrence is at least ten times the reported numbers, but projections from the Council for Agricultural Science and Technology are as high as 33 million cases of food poisoning annually. Other reports range as high as 80 million.

Food contamination means that a food has levels of microbes that create a potential risk to human health, and can occur during growing, shipping, improper refrigeration (the number-one source of contamination), or processing. Meats, for example, may be infected even before the animals are slaughtered. **Food poisoning** is the

SOURCES OF CONTAMINATION DURING PRODUCTION

Phase	Sources

Production and harvest
    Growing, picking, bundling
	Irrigation water, manure, lack of field
	    sanitation

Initial processing
    Washing, waxing, sorting,
    boxing
	Wash water, handling, inadequate
	    hygiene of environment, pests

Distribution Transport by truck, rail, or sea	Ice, dirty trucks, or tankers

Final processing
    Slicing, squeezing, shredding,
    peeling, mechanical extraction,
    mixing of batches
	Wash water, handling, poor hygiene
	    of equipment, cross-contamination

Display in the supermarket
    Handling, moisturizing, displaying
	Inadequate hygiene of employees, cross
	    contamination in displays, infested
	    produce sprays, airborne microbes

sickness that people experience, mainly from exposure to bacteria and viruses. It is estimated that about 9,000 people die each year from food-related contamination—about 25 people a day. However, only about 1,000 deaths a year are documented. Taking specific precautions when we prepare food at home helps to minimize contamination by microorganisms such as bacteria, viruses, protozoa, or molds.

Contamination of the human digestive tract by microscopic parasites, pathogenic bacteria, or viruses is most often the cause of acute diarrhea. The FDA points out that some people are more at risk than others, and the choice and preparation of their foods requires greater care. Those most at risk include:

- Children and infants
- Pregnant women
- Older adults

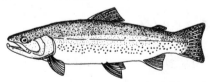

- People with weakened immune systems, such as those with HIV, AIDS, or cancer
- People on acid blockers or who have low stomach acid output, because stomach acid offers natural protection against microbes.

Bacterial Food Poisonings

A 1982 study of traceable cases of food poisoning found that more than half were caused by contaminated poultry and seafood (about 20% chicken and 40% fish), mainly shellfish. Only about 10% involved viruses. Currently, salmonella, shigella, and campylobacter are the common bacteria that cause food poisoning. They infect animals and are then passed on to humans in our food. Other less common illnesses are important because, although rare, they can be fatal. These include E. coli, listeria, and botulism (caused by the *Clostridium botulinum* bacteria). All of these bacterial infections usually require medical intervention, and antibiotics have helped many sufferers to recover.

• **Salmonella** infection comes most commonly from contaminated animal protein that is improperly cooked, such as raw milk and unpasteurized cheeses; undercooked meat, poultry, fish, and eggs; products made with eggs, such as mayonnaise; unpasteurized juices; and contaminated sprouts. There are an estimated 2 to 3 million cases in the U.S. each year of undiagnosed salmonella food poisoning, although most of these are mild to moderate infections. Food poisoning from salmonella produces fever, chills, diarrhea, abdominal pain, sometimes vomiting, and often a severe headache. Fortunately, it is rarely fatal and will respond to treatment with an antibiotic such as ampicillin. Symptoms usually clear in 1 to 2 days.

It has been suggested that the increased bacterial contamination in meat is due mainly to lack of hygiene in factory farming environments. This is a good reason to moderate your intake of animal protein and to buy organic meats whenever possible. **In general, salmonella can best be avoided by thoroughly cooking all dishes that include meat, poultry, seafood, or eggs and by using only pasteurized milks and cheeses.** Although these foods are usually safe in the uncooked or unpasteurized state, they are more easily contaminated with salmonella than other foods.

• **Campylobacter** is another bacterial illness originating in poultry, and which can cause diarrhea, cramping, pain, and fever about 2 to 5 days after exposure. Over 10,000 cases are reported to the CDC each year, and it also estimates that it may actually affect as many as 2 million people each year, about 1% of the population. It occurs more frequently in the summer, and more often to infants and young adults. It is fatal in about 500 cases a year.

Poultry is typically the source of campylobacter in 99% of cases; birds can carry it without becoming ill. *So the best way to avoid this infection is to cook all poultry thoroughly.*

• **Shigella** is a group of bacteria that also cause gastrointestinal illness, with symptoms of fever, abdominal pain, and diarrhea. The bacteria is transmitted through direct contact, through food handled by someone with an infection, and through contaminated water. It most commonly affects milk and dairy products, poultry, tuna, shrimp, and raw vegetables. In 1995, more than 32,000 cases were reported to the CDC, almost double the number 10 years earlier. It can be fatal in about 10% of cases. Children and food handlers are most frequently the carriers. **The single most important way to prevent shigellosis is hand washing with antibacterial soap and clean, running water.** It is essential to teach our children to wash their hands thoroughly and consistently, and to follow through with monitoring and guidance to protect their health.

• **E. coli** is another bacterial illness. The strain O157:H7 is an emerging cause of foodborne illness. Although only about 2,000 cases were reported in 1995, it is estimated that more than 20,000 cases of infection occur in the U.S. each year. Problems may be severe, including bloody diarrhea and occasionally kidney failure and fatality. The primary cause to date is undercooked beef. It can also come from drinking contaminated raw milk, unpasteurized fruit juices, and sewage-contaminated water. It can be transmitted through person-to-person contact in families and in child care centers. Since most cases of E. coli have been associated with eating undercooked ground beef, **the primary prevention includes cooking beef and hamburger to at least 160°F on the meat thermometer.**

• **Listeria** is a less common, but quite serious bacterial infection. Listeria is the bacteria that can cause meningitis, a serious illness that can result in brain injury or death. Although only an estimated 2,000 cases are reported each year, of these 425 (over 20%) are fatal. Listeria primarily affects those most vulnerable, particularly pregnant women and people with AIDS, and typically begins with flulike symptoms.

This bacteria is found in soil and water and as a contaminant in manure. Listeria is contracted from raw foods—raw or uncooked meats, hot dogs, poultry, and fish; occasionally in raw vegetables or ice cream; in raw milk, unpasteurized cheeses (camembert, brie, or Mexican style cheese); and contaminated processed foods such as deli cold cuts. **The best way to prevent this life-threatening infection is to avoid any listeria contaminated foods.**

• **Botulism** is a rare but serious foodborne disease, caused by the contamination of food from *Clostridium botulinum* bacteria commonly found in the soil. Botulism toxins are most frequently transmitted in spoiled, home-canned food, and occasionally in contaminated fish and other commercial food products. Botulism in infants is caused by eating the spores of botulinum bacteria, in sources such as honey. Although there are only about 100 cases a year in the U.S., botulism can be fatal. The botulism toxin is destroyed by boiling for 10 minutes, so home-canned food is safest if boiled. **The FDA recommends that children less than a year old not be fed honey and that careful precautions are taken in home canning and the use of home-canned foods.**

Other Foodborne Infections

• **Hepatitis A, known as infectious hepatitis,** is usually transmitted by human carriers, including agricultural fieldworkers, workers in food processing factories, or by those who handle and prepare foods at home or in restaurants. Shellfish and strawberries have been found to be contaminated with the hepatitis virus. Most intestinal viruses (and bacteria) are typically transferred from the hands, *so hand washing is the best way to prevent transmitting this and other infectious agents.*

• **Amoebas** represent one of the most common worldwide parasitic problems, and a potential food- and waterborne organism. As *Entamoeba histolyica* and other Entamoeba species, they cause a range of symptoms from acute dysentery with fever, chills, and pain to mild persistent or episodic indigestion. People who handle or prepare food can pass it to others, much like infectious hepatitis. *Washing hands and scrubbing fingernails with soap and water before handling food is an important step for preventing amoebas, as is true with most foodborne infections.*

• **Molds** are the most common microbes that contaminate foods. They can grow on cheeses, breads, meats, herbs, nuts, or grains. In general, most molds are fairly well tolerated when consumed in small amounts. Some people, however, are allergic or sensitive to molds. Also, certain molds found on specific foods may produce toxins that can cause serious illness. Aflatoxin, produced by the molds *Aspergillus flavus* and *parasiticus*, is potentially harmful, especially to the liver, where it can cause a type of hepatitis or even cancer. It has been associated most commonly with peanuts but can also contaminate other nuts, as well as corn, wheat, and barley.

Like molds, many bacteria produce toxins, and certain shellfish and mushrooms contain toxic chemicals that can cause intestinal upset and even fatal neurotoxicity. Bread and cheese molds may cause some allergic-type reactions, but these agents are generally less harmful. **To prevent molding of your foods, buy them fresh, store them well, and refrigerate or freeze them if you are not using them soon.**

• **Cryptosporidium** is a potential foodborne problem from contaminated water. Enough concentrations of this parasite may cause symptoms in anyone, as shown during an epidemic seven years ago in Milwaukee where thousands were hospitalized from contaminated water. **Filtering water is the best way to protect against cryptosporidium.**

How Do You Know If You Have Food Poisoning?

One answer is, of course, you'll know! The most typical symptoms are diarrhea (the body's attempt to shed the offending organisms), abdominal cramping, and fever, as well as headache, vomiting, and severe exhaustion. These and other symptoms may develop as quickly as 30 minutes after eating or may take days or weeks to occur (with listeria, for example). Food poisoning can last from 6 to 12 hours up to a week or so before things settle back to normal.

IT'S TIME TO CALL THE DOCTOR WHEN YOU HAVE:

- **A fever above 102°:** This may indicate a serious infection or a simple flu.
- **Bloody diarrhea:** This is a sign of possible E. coli infection.
- **A stiff neck, severe headache, and fever:** All three occuring at once could be a sign of meningitis (an inflammation of the brain lining) caused by listeria.
- **Excessive diarrhea or vomiting:** This could lead to life-threatening dehydration. You are probably dehydrated if you haven't urinated in 12 hours.
- **Any food poisoning symptoms that last for more than 3 days.**

Here are a few ideas for natural therapy support if you become ill from contaminated food or water. Begin by replacing fluids, especially if you are feverish, vomiting, or have diarrhea. Also, you can support your digestive tract with hourly doses

	FOOD CONTAMINATION BY MICROBES		
Microbe	**Source**	**Reported Cases '95**	**Estimated Cases '95**
Bacteria			
Botulism	Spoiled home-canned foods; spores in honey; contaminated fish	97	—
Campylobacter	Undercooked poultry, especially giblets and chicken livers; raw milk	10,000+	2,000,000+
E. coli	Meat, unpasteurized fruit juices, and raw milk	2,139	20,000
Listeria (causes meningitis)	Undercooked meat, poultry, pork; water; unpasteurized soft cheeses; raw milk; in vegetables, but rare	1,600* (Fatal 415*)	1,850
Salmonella	Undercooked poultry, beef, fish; uncooked eggs in eggnog, etc. undercooked omelets, quiches, etc; unpasteurized juices; sprouts	45,970	637,000 to 1,000,000+
Shigella	Transmitted by food handlers; deli salads: potato, tuna, shrimp; milk and dairy products; poultry; raw vegetables	32,080	300,000
Vibrio (cholera)	Shellfish; oysters and clams	23	Unknown[c]
Yersinia	Meats, oysters, fish; raw milk	—	17,000

of 500 to 1,000 mg L-glutamine, along with 1 to 2 capsules of a probiotic formula (healthy bacteria—*Lactobacillus acidophilus* and *Bifidobacteria,* the two most common, are available at most health food stores) while waiting for the doctor at home or in the emergency room. Since antibiotics and other medications can take a little while to become effective, the use of probiotics and L-glutamine is an excellent complement to any appropriate drug therapy.

Given all the concerns, it is helpful to know that our society has coped successfully with such problems in the past. Typhoid fever, which was very common at the beginning of the twentieth century, is now almost forgotten in the United States. It was conquered in the preantibiotic era through the treatment of water and sewage,

Microscopic Parasites

Amoebas (e.g. E. histolytica)	Food handlers; sexual contact; drinking water; some foods	3,328**	2,000,000+
Blastocystis	Food handlers; food and water	Not yet tracked	
Cryptosporidium	Drinking water; fruit or juices; sometimes raw vegetables	—	5,000,000+
Cyclospora	Contaminated food and water	—	Rare/serious
Giardia	Drinking water	—	2,000,000
Trichinosis	Undercooked pork	2	—

Viruses

Hepatitis A	Food handlers; contaminated water or foods (such as shellfish or salads)	31,582	—
Norwalk-virus	Food handlers; Raw/undercooked oysters or clams		Frequent

Natural Toxins

Aflatoxins (Aspergillis mold)	Peanuts and other nuts; corn, cottonseed, milk	Unknown[c]	
Ciguatera toxin	Large finfish: jack, mackerel; large grouper and snapper	Unknown[c]	
Mushroom toxins	Specific toxic species of mushrooms	44 cases in 5 years	Rare, but can be fatal
Shellfish poisoning	Potentially any shellfish: mussels, clams, oysters, scallops	Unknown[c]	Rare, but can be fatal

Sources: Centers for Disease Control, "Summary of Notifiable Diseases (1995)"
Morbidity and Mortality Report (MMWR) 44(53): 1996 October 25.
and other data from the Centers for Disease Control web site at <www.cdc.gov>
* Data from 1987   ** Data from 1990   [c] Quoted from the Centers for Disease Control

the pasteurization of milk, and improved shellfish sanitation. Similarly, cholera, bovine tuberculosis, and trichinosis have also been successfully controlled in this country. **Note that the suggested preventive strategies in this chapter can reduce the microbial content in food and water.** Today, in what many are calling the postantibiotic era when many microbes are developing drug resistance, it is essential that we return to hygiene and other common sense approaches to avoid illness.

AVOIDING FOODBORNE INFECTIONS

Did you know that the CDC found that the main cause of food poisoning is storing or preparing food at the wrong temperature? This caused a third of all the outbreaks from 1988 to 1992. Also, they found that poor hygiene and unsafe food sources accounted for more than a quarter of the outbreaks of food poisoning.

Although you can't control the temperature at which food is stored before you buy it, there are things you *can* do to insure that you are buying food that has been handled properly. Shop at a store you trust—one that buys from reputable sources. And make sure that your market is as clean as possible. (Remember—as the consumer, you have a choice.) Are they impeccable in their handling of seafood and meats? Don't buy or use bulging cans, outdated foods, or packaged foods with broken seals. Avoid buying overly ripe produce. Beware of buying from roadside vendors, and avoid purchasing eggs sitting out in flats, unrefrigerated. The fish at outdoor markets or roadside stands may look good, but you don't know how it was handled or how clean the ice is that it was packed in. Ask questions, and trust your powers of observation and your intuition. It's not worth the risk of becoming sick.

Once you purchase your groceries, it becomes your job to control their storage temperature. Don't leave food sitting in a hot car. **Remember that animal proteins are most often the source of food poisoning—that means poultry, fish, meat, eggs, and unpasteurized cheeses. Refrigerate meats, poultry, and seafood immediately and use them within 2 days, or freeze them as soon as you get home from shopping. Frozen foods should be kept frozen, defrosted in the fridge (not on the counter), and used soon after thawing.**

Cleanliness in the Kitchen

Once antibiotics were developed, some people began taking hygiene less seriously. It was felt that any bacterial infection could be easily treated, so why worry? But now we know that antibiotics should be reserved for major illnesses and that prevention of disease is always the ideal approach. Safe practices in the kitchen afford us this preventive protection, but they require a return to the kind of organization and planning that our grandparents used. For example, soaking salad vegetables in order to avoid microbes and clean off pesticides requires 20 minutes. So, if we know that we are going to use raw vegetables in our dinner salad, for example, we need to fit those 20 minutes into our routine. We can either get into washing salad

SHOPPING SAFETY CHECKLIST

❏ Read labels to minimize the risk of food poisoning. Check the product dating for freshness.

❏ Buy only those milk and cheese products that are pasteurized. Avoid unpasteurized cheeses such as brie, Camembert, blue-veined cheeses, etc.

❏ Buy only ciders and juices that are pasteurized.

❏ Don't buy eggs that are unrefrigerated—for example, eggs sitting out at roadside stands. And be sure to put eggs in the refrigerator as soon as you get home. (The FDA found that merely keeping eggs cold enough cut bacteria by 25%.)

❏ Avoid prepared foods that contain raw or partially cooked meat or dairy products.

❏ Avoid potatoes that are green-skinned or have developed eyes and sprouts.

❏ Bag all vegetables before going through the checkout to avoid bacteria at the counters.

❏ Place protein foods (chicken, eggs, fish, and meat) into a plastic bag to prevent leakage of uncooked eggs or meat juices onto other foods, which causes cross-contamination (the transmission of bacteria from one food to another).

❏ Avoid potentially contaminated foods: foods in damaged packaging; foods displayed unsafely, such as cooked and uncooked seafood on the same bed of ice; free food samples, open air displays of perishable food, and salad bars are more risky for contamination; or foods found in stores with unsanitary conditions.

❏ When transporting your groceries, keep perishables inside the air-conditioned car, not the trunk.

❏ If you live more than a half an hour from the store, bring an ice chest for storing perishables on the way home.

❏ Refrigerate or freeze perishables immediately. Keep the refrigerator temperature at 40°F and the freezer at 0°F.

❏ Remember that chicken and fish need to be cooked the first or second day. So during the holidays, if you must buy fish or poultry ahead, get it frozen. Fresh, unfrozen turkey needs to be bought just a day or two before cooking.

❏ Put protein foods in your shopping cart last, so they stay as cold as possible.

❏ Put chilled or frozen items in the shopping cart last, right before you head for the checkout line.

veggies as soon as we come home from the store, or figure those extra minutes into our food preparation time.

Washing our hands before working in the kitchen is a basic cleanliness ritual, but one that we sometimes neglect. **It is essential that everybody who handles food take responsibility for keeping their hands clean.** You should wash your hands before working with food, especially after going to the bathroom, handling animals or money or anything handled by others, or caring for children, particularly after wiping their noses or changing diapers. (For example, unusually high rates of giardia infection occur in daycare centers, due to transmission through diaper changing and personal contact.) Hands should be washed with an antibacterial soap and warm water, and nails should be brushed with soap or hydrogen peroxide. You should also avoid handling foods when you are sick. If there are cuts or open sores on your hands, rubber gloves will reduce the spread of bacteria.

Surfaces, such as kitchen countertops and cutting boards, should be cleaned after each use so that organisms don't grow. Cutting utensils should also be spotlessly clean. Sponges should be cleaned (run through the dishwasher or zapped in the microwave) and replaced frequently. Can openers need to be cleaned regularly as well, and replaced occasionally. Pots and pans, blenders, and juicers need thorough cleaning after each use.

More food poisoning occurs at home than in restaurants! But that means we have a measure of control over our own health. Read ahead for more tips on keeping food and kitchen areas sparkling clean.

Guidelines for Keeping a Safe and Clean Kitchen

- If you're sick, if at all possible, don't cook. Food handling is a major way in which germs get transmitted. If you must cook, wear disposable gloves, or if you are coughing or sneezing, consider wearing a mask.
- Keep your shelves, drawers, countertops, refrigerator, freezer, and utensils really clean.
- Wipe the tops of cans before opening to prevent germ contamination.
- Wipe countertops with hot water and soap and then with a disinfectant (preferably a safe cleaner, such as an antibacterial soap, a diluted bleach solution, or vinegar and water)
- Clean the drain of the kitchen sink weekly by pouring in a solution of 1 teaspoon bleach to 1 quart of water.

- Clean kitchen equipment thoroughly. On holidays or at other times, when using stored equipment, clean it thoroughly before and after use.
- If you hand wash the dishes, do them within two hours after they've been used. Don't let them soak for a long period, which creates a "bacterial soup." And use very warm water. If you use a dishwasher, run it with hot water.
- Wash towels often on the hot water cycle. Wash sponges in the dish washer or zap them in the microwave for 30 to 60 seconds to kill germs. Or use disposable, recycled paper towels. Most sponges are made with and contain chemicals.
- Wash your hands in soap and warm water for 20 seconds before and after handling food. *You'll find that 20 seconds is an amazingly long time—but it's important!*
- Wash your hands every time you change the baby, use the bathroom, or blow your nose.
- Wash your hands thoroughly after handling pets, and before cooking or handling food. Animals harbor many microbes harmful to humans. This is true of cats and dogs, reptiles and especially turtles (which carry listeria). Many cats, for example, carry H. pylori (one of the major causes of ulcers) and toxoplasmosis (devastating to the unborn).
- After using the bathroom, scrub under your nails with a brush dipped in hydrogen peroxide. This can prevent the transfer of bacteria and the cysts (containing eggs) of microscopic parasites, which tend to lodge under the fingernails.
- Avoid cross-contamination. Wash up after handling one food, and before handling the next. This is especially important if you are handling raw protein such as chicken, fish, meat, or eggs. It also minimizes the contamination of other foods that won't be cooked, such as salads.
- It is ideal to have two cutting boards, one for meat and the other for vegetables. Save wooden boards made of hard maple for use with your produce.
- Use plastic cutting boards for preparing protein foods (chicken, fish, and meat). Research shows that plastic boards collect less bacteria. Replace the plastic boards when they become scored by knife abrasion, since bacteria can collect on the uneven surface.
- Be sure to clean all cutting boards with soap, hot water, and a bleach solution (1 teaspoon to 1 quart of hot water). Soak the surface for several minutes, then dry it thoroughly. Or wash it in the dishwasher.

- After food is cooked, care must also be taken to avoid contamination. Bacteria reproduce rapidly at room temperature. *Do not let foods sit out overnight.*

Cleaning Methods to Reduce Exposure to Germs and Chemicals

Since about two-thirds of all nonorganic produce typically contains pesticide residues, and since organic and nonorganically grown foods may be contaminated with insect eggs or germs such as E. coli or cyclospora, it is wise to wash all fresh produce thoroughly. **The outer layer on all nonorganic produce should be discarded: peel fruits and strip the outer leaves of cabbage, lettuces, and other leafy greens. Wash your produce thoroughly in running water. Researchers have found that just rinsing lettuce, for example, isn't enough to get rid of the bacteria. Washing the leaves individually is more effective.**

To be extra safe, wash produce with natural disinfectants (see following discussion) that may clean off additional surface chemicals and pesticides. All produce, even organically grown foods, can harbor microbes. The lack of chemicals in organic produce may allow even more bacteria and pests to inhabit it. Therefore, to be safe from microbial food contamination, wash everything—organic and nonorganic produce alike.

In the past, I have recommended washing your produce with vinegar and water, produce soaps, or diluted chlorine bleach. Tests reported in *Consumer Reports* reveal that this appears to remove about 50% of the pesticide residues, if the residues are on the surface. However, produce washed in this manner often has an unpleasant aftertaste. **A solution of bleach, 1 or so teaspoons to 2 quarts of water, can be used to soak leafy greens. This should take 15 to 20 minutes. Then soak and rinse the greens thoroughly in clean water. However, this too can leave an aftertaste.**

In recent years, several improved, naturally-derived produce washes have become available: EarthSafe, OrganiClean, and VegiWash. These rinses and sprays act as natural detergents to remove some of the pesticides and dirt. Most of these cleansing agents are made from fruit or vegetable and coconut extracts, are sprayed on fruits and vegetables, and then rinsed off with water. These seem to be safer and better ways to be protected from foodborne illnesses. They are designed to wash off surface contaminants, both chemicals and germs. However, they cannot remove "systemic" pesticides, those that are in the tissue and fiber of the plant and can't be removed with surface cleaning. **To avoid systemic insecticides, our best option is to buy organically grown produce instead.**

Although most of us would prefer to use plain water to rinse our vegetables, toxicologists report that some pesticides do stick to produce, making a detergent cleansing necessary. Since E. coli can live in manure for as long as 70 days, and can multiply in foods grown in manure, it is helpful to soak our vegetables thoroughly to remove bacteria.

Generic testing reported by National Resource Defense Council (NRDC) indicates that some nonsystemic pesticides tend to stick to the surface and are more thoroughly removed with a detergent-like product. Testing by Consumers Union recently found that a diluted wash of dish detergent, followed by a tap water rinse, reduced pesticide residues to zero in about half the samples tested. However, since small residues of the detergent probably cling to the produce, the concern here is that most dish detergents are not designed for human consumption, and contain their own chemicals, colors, and perfumes.

The organic cleansers are promising, because they are made for this purpose from food-based products. However, these are costly, and without actual testing data, we must withhold judgment on any specific claims made by manufacturers.

COOKING METHODS AND MAINTAINING NUTRITION

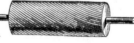

After food is cooked, care must also be taken to avoid contamination. Bacteria that are usually destroyed in cooking grow very slowly when cold, but multiply rapidly at room temperature. Cooked foods should not be left sitting out overnight. Also, if you do any home canning, be sure to do it under extremely clean conditions; when done improperly, this is the most common cause of botulism (meats and green beans being the worst culprits).

The primary cooking procedures most of us use include boiling, steaming, baking, sautéing, frying, and grilling/barbecuing. Slow cookers and crock pots are also popular. Let's review these briefly and see how they stack up in terms of both avoiding microbial contamination and retaining nutrients. Basically, all cooking methods reduce or eradicate germs (see Cooking Temperature next).

COOKING TEMPERATURES TO MINIMIZE RISK

Food	Temperature	Risks
Eggs: cook thoroughly. Avoid raw eggs in any form like eggnog. Avoid lightly cooked eggs in omelets, French toast, Caesar salad, hollandaise sauce, mousse, meringue pie, quiche	Cook to 160°F—until not runny Scrambled: 1 min. med. (250°F) Sunnyside: 7 min. med.; 4 min. covered Fried: 3 min. first side, 1 min. over Poached: 5 min. in boiling water Boiled: 7 min. in boiling water	Listeria Salmonella
Beef, veal, lamb Ground beef, ham: Meats, medium: Meats, well-done:	Avoid all raw meats & dishes— beefsteak tartar 160°F 160°F 170°F	E. coli Listeria Salmonella
Pork Ham	Cook to 160°F to 170°F Cook at 160°F; if the ham is precooked 140°F	Listeria Trichinosis

Poultry
   Chicken or turkey, ground
   Chicken or turkey, whole
   Breasts, roasts
   Thighs, wings
	Cook to at least:
	165°F
	180°F
	170°F
	Cook until juices run clear
		Cyclospora
		Camplobacter
		Listeria
		Salmonella

Fish and Seafood	Cook well; until flaky, not rubbery Cook seafood well: Avoid sushi, sashimi; Note source of seafood	Botulism Cholera, Listeria, Staph, Vibrio

Shellfish: Clams, Cockles,
Mussels, Oysters, Scallops
	Cook well: Avoid lightly steamed
	    seafood; seafood can no longer
	    safely be eaten raw
		Hepatitis A

Leftovers	165°F; meats in 200°F oven; warming tray 140°F	Any bacteria

Boiling

Whole grains, beans, hot cereals, soups, and eggs are often boiled or, preferably, simmered slowly. I cook grains such as brown rice, millet, and buckwheat by bringing water to a boil and adding the grain (1 part to 2 parts water). I simmer or slowly boil for 20 to 40 minutes until the grain is cooked. Beans take longer. We want as much nutrition as possible to stay in the food; however, we will lose some water-soluble vitamins, such as the Bs and C, when we boil. Still, boiled foods will retain any fat-soluble vitamins and much of their minerals.

Steaming

When we steam food, many of the nutrients will go into the steam and then drip back into the water. Therefore, the liquid, or "pot liquor," could be more nourishing than the food. This will occur less if we use larger-cut steaming vegetables, if we don't overcook, or if we steam proteins that have a skin or outer coating, such as hot dogs made of chicken, beef, or tofu (free of nitrites, of course). Steaming is a very simple and efficient way to make and eat vegetables, and many people find them easier to digest this way. To kill germs, steam for 15 minutes.

Baking

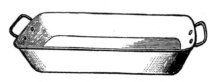

This is a safe way to cook animal proteins, and an easy way to prepare vegetables. Allowing food to cook thoroughly at 300° to 400°F will kill any microbes. Salmon and chicken are ideally baked in a covered dish. I usually add some oil or butter and seasonings, a few tablespoons of water to keep it juicy, and chopped onions, garlic, carrots, and potatoes to bake in the same dish. Or I may put some potatoes in the oven alongside my baking dish. We can conserve energy when we cook everything together. Baking is an excellent way to assure that nutrients remain in the food.

Sautéing (or Stir-frying)

One of my favorite cooking methods I call water-sautéing or stir-frying. I use a hot iron skillet and small amounts of olive or canola oil to coat the pan first, then add a little more oil at the end for essential fatty acids and more flavor. I use small amounts of water as I cook so that the steam and the flavors permeate the foods. I love cooking vegetables and tofu this way, combining onions, carrots, mushrooms, snow peas, broccoli, zucchini, and whatever other vegetables appeal to me. There are also a variety of prepared tofu dishes already made with added sauces (usually available in the coolers in the natural food store or natural foods section) that can be sautéed with vegetables and served over rice. Nutritionally speaking, this combination of tofu, rice, and veggies is just about as good as it gets.

The sautéing or stir-frying method really is as nutritious as it appears. A study at Tufts University on the benefits of stir-frying compared nutrients in food cooked by boiling, microwaving, and stir-frying. Stir-fried food did well, with the highest levels of nutrients (vitamin C) remaining in cooked broccoli.

Slow-cooking

This method can be a real convenience when making soups, chili, stews, or spaghetti sauces. Cut the food into chunks or small pieces to be sure it cooks thoroughly. Don't use your slow cooker for large pieces of meat or a whole chicken because the meat will cook too slowly and the bacteria may not be totally destroyed. If possible, turn the cooker on high for the first hour and then turn to a lower setting. This is a great way to cook grains and beans, and it retains most of the nutrients.

Frying

This cooking process (involving a full oil sauté or deep frying) can add significant fat calories to your meal. When cooking with heated oils, it's best to use monounsaturated oils, such as olive or canola oil, and limit the use of polyunsaturates, such as corn or safflower oils, which are less stable under heat. Deep-fried foods should only be eaten as occasional treats, and then followed by appropriate antioxidants, including vitamins E and C, and beta-carotene.

Grilling/Barbecuing

This can be a tasty way to prepare vegetables, meats, and other proteins. Grilling is similar to broiling, with a high heat directly adjacent to the food. Many restaurants now offer grilled foods in a process very similar to a barbecue, as in mesquite grilling. Most people barbecue primarily animal proteins, and care must be taken to cook them thoroughly enough to eradicate bacteria. Other health concerns include charcoal toxins and lighter fluids, so the best grilling option appears to be the use of propane gas grills, which can cook foods thoroughly. The new, fancy grills can even be programmed to cook foods to specific temperatures and times. I like to grill vegetables on the barbecue, such as zucchini strips coated lightly with

WATER SOLUBLE VITAMINS IN FOODS (VEGETABLES & POULTRY)

Average Percentage after Various Cooking Methods

	Vitamin C in Vegetables		B Vitamins in Poultry	
Cooking method	Broccoli	Green beans	Thiamine	Riboflavin
Braising/simmering	74%	76%	64%	93%
Stir-frying	77%	58%		
Microwave	57%	59%	64%	94%
Frying			46%	79%
Boiling–much water		45%	60%	
Roasting			29%	60%

Source: *International Journal of Food Sciences and Nutrition*, March 1988.

olive oil, corn, eggplant, bell peppers, and garlic. Grilled vegetables are very tasty—and they do best on a barbecue with a cover to allow full cooking heat. Also, grilled and barbecued foods retain much of their nutrition.

Some people like to cook food partially on the stove or in the microwave to cut down on grilling time. If you do this, precook your food immediately before grilling. Then grill it until it reaches a safe temperature. Other people like to partially grill meat and then refrigerate or freeze it and finish cooking it at a later time. Storing partially cooked food, even in the freezer, isn't recommended, however, because when food is only partly cooked, the bacteria aren't thoroughly destroyed.

Microwaving

Microwave ovens appear to be relatively nontoxic when used occasionally and if you don't stand too close to them while they're on. My family uses the microwave primarily to reheat leftovers. Microwaves use pico waves, which penetrate tissue deeply and rapidly, and increase the vibrational rate of the water and tissue molecules. This process generates the heat and cooks the food. Being too close to an active microwave oven can result in symptoms such as headaches, fatigue, irritability, sleeping problems, and even tissue burns. Such symptoms have been noted in restaurant workers who use microwave ovens regularly. Continuous microwave cooking exposure may also cause hormonal changes and affect our immune defenses, and the long-term effects are not yet known. These ovens are a great convenience, but we shouldn't be dependent on them. Also, remember that packaging on microwaveable foods can contaminate food at high temperatures. So use only microwave-safe containers.

AVOIDING FOOD CONTAMINATION

Food	Prevention of Infection	Risk
Milk, raw	Purchase only pasteurized milk	Campylobacter, E. Coli, Listeria, Salmonella
Raw cheeses: Brie, blue-veined, Camembert, feta	To be avoided by infants, children, elders, and those with chronic illness	Listeria
Water	Filter to "1 micron absolute" or boil for 15 minutes	Campylobacter, Cryptosporidium, E. Coli, Giardia
Honey	Do not feed to infants or those who are immuno-compromised	Botulism
Fruit juices, Cider	Buy pasteurized or bring to a boil	E. coli
Fruits: Cantaloupe, Raspberries, Strawberries, frozen	Wash thoroughly; soak in OrganoClean or other natural disenfectant	Salmonella, Cyclospora, Hepatitis A
Vegetables and Tomatoes	Soak in OrganoClean or water with 1 teaspoon bleach	Cyclospora, E. Coli, Listeria, Salmonella, Shigella
Home canning— avoiding spoilage from storage	Boil for 10 minutes at above 165°F	Botulism
Spices: Paprika	Store in refrigerator	Salmonella

Source: FDA

Cooking Safely

One of the primary reasons we cook food is to sanitize it. Remember that heat kills bacteria. But the food has to be hot enough throughout, at least 160° to 180°F.

Meat, Poultry, and Fish

- If you want to make certain that bacteria or microscopic parasites are killed in the process of cooking, **never cook meat, chicken, or fish for less than 20 minutes**. No pink should exist (except turkey and smoked meats, which will continue to appear pink, despite their thermometer temperature). Use the meat temperature, 160° to 170°F, to be sure when foods are well done. Juices should run clear, not red.
- When roasting meat and poultry, use an oven temperature no lower than 325°F.
- Do not refrigerate or freeze partially cooked meat, poultry, or fish.
- Thaw animal proteins in the refrigerator rather than on the counter. This can take some planning—a 20-pound turkey needs a couple days to thaw in the fridge!
- Frozen foods can also be thawed more quickly by wrapping them in a sealed plastic bag, submerging them in cold tap water, and changing the water every 30 minutes so it stays cold. Then cook immediately after thawing or refrigerate.
- Thaw animal foods thoroughly, so they can cook all the way through.
- Marinate meat and poultry in a covered dish in the refrigerator.
- Use a meat thermometer to be sure protein foods are thoroughly cooked—it could save your life!
- Use a conventional meat thermometer; it gives you more information than a pop-up thermometer.
- If you're making stuffing, cook it separately from the chicken or turkey, on the stovetop, or in the oven. If you must cook it inside the bird, stuff it just before baking and make sure the stuffing reaches 165°F on the meat thermometer.
- When baking fish, compute the baking time based on at least 10 minutes per inch of thickness at the thickest part of the fish. Bake at 450°F in a preheated oven. You can bake at 350 to 400° F, but it takes longer. I often do this when I add vegetables to the baking dish with the fish.
- Since fish exposed to water chemicals store them primarily in their fat and skin, cut away any excess fat to lower your potential exposure. This is also true of other animal fats, as in meats and poultry.

Eggs and Egg Dishes

- Pasteurized eggs can be used in place of raw eggs to make homemade ice cream, eggnog, caesar salad dressing, mayonnaise, and hollandaise sauce. Commercial versions of these products are okay because they're made with pasteurized liquid eggs.
- If you want to pasteurize the eggs yourself, heat the egg-milk mixture to 160°F (until it coats a metal spoon). When you don't have time to make or buy pasteurized eggs, leave them out of recipes that don't involve baking or cooking, rather than take a chance.
- Do not eat cookie batter that contains uncooked eggs. (If you find the dough irresistible, make or buy pasteurized eggs for the batter.)
- Keep eggs in the refrigerator below 40°F. Cook them at 140°F or hotter.
- When cooking eggs, make sure the yolk and white are firm, not runny. Eggs need to be cooked on both sides, rather than just sunny-side up. Cook scrambled eggs until firm.) If you're served runny eggs in a restaurant, send them back—*it's your health!*)
- Avoid keeping raw or cooked eggs or egg dishes out of the refrigerator for more than 2 hours. Easter eggs should be refrigerated after 2 hours or considered decoration only.
- When refrigerating a dish made with eggs, divide it and store it in several shallow containers so it will cool throughout.

Leftovers and Convenience Foods

- Don't taste food to be sure that it's still good. There may be no sign that it's spoiled.
- If a food smells or tastes spoiled, return it to the store or throw it out.
- Boil leftover soups, sauces, and gravies.
- Thoroughly reheat leftovers, at least to 165°F, or until hot and steamy.
- Use leftovers within 4 days.
- If you're microwaving your food, follow the directions carefully. Since the goal is to cook protein foods thoroughly, be sure to include the "standard time" that some microwave recipes suggest. This is also part of the cooking process.

Serving Food Safely

Bacteria thrive in the same environments we do—at room temperature. So keep food very hot or very cold from kitchen to table.

- Serve cooked foods as soon as they're ready.
- To avoid bacteria increases, never leave food out longer than 2 hours.

NONTOXIC HOUSEHOLD CLEANERS

Products	Concerns	Best Option
Dishwashing liquid	May have dye, ammonia, artificial fragrance	"Green" products
Dishwasher detergent	Chlorine	Green products now in health food stores: Seventh Generation products available through mail order
Cleanser	Chlorine; Possible asbestos	Nonchlorinated scouring powder; available in supermarkets & health food stores; baking soda, borax, salt
Germ-killing disinfectants	Cresol, phenol, ethanol, formaldehyde, ammonia, chlorine	1/2 cup borax in 1 gallon hot water; hydrogen peroxide; solution of benzalkonium chloride
Drain cleaners	Lye (poisonous)	1 handful baking soda & 1/2 cup white vinegar or 1/2 cup each salt & baking soda followed by hot water. Follow by using plunger
Ammonia & all-purpose cleaners	Ammonia (skin irritant, chemical burns); aerosol sprays	1 quart hot water in a spray bottle or bucket with either liquid soap or borax; or green products
Chlorine bleach	Chlorine byproducts	Nonchlorine bleach (Seventh Generation)
Cleaners for appliances		1/2 t. washing soda, 2 t. liquid soap & 2 cups hot water
Oven cleaner	Lye, ammonia, aerosols	Use chemicals carefully for really dirty ovens; or in a spray bottle, add 2 T. liquid soap, 2 t. borax, warm water; or make a paste of liq. soap & borax
Glass cleaners	Ammonia, blue dye, aerosol	Solution of half water & half vinegar in spray bottle or bucket
Mold & mildew cleaners	Kerosene, formaldehyde, phenol, pentachloro-phenol	Borax or vinegar & water Heat and/or dehumidifier

Source: Courtesy of Debra Lynn Dadd, *The Nontoxic Home & Office* (1992) and *Home, Safe Home* (1996) Tarcher / Putnam, New York.

- On a hot day, over 90°F, don't leave food out longer than 1 hour.
- When serving food at a buffet, keep hot food over a heat source and keep cold food on ice.
- Keep platters of food refrigerated until it's time to serve or heat them.
- Don't serve all the food at once. Keep the second and third servings hot in the oven (above 140°F) or cold in the refrigerator (below 40°F).
- When you serve later courses, put the food on clean platters, instead of adding it to platters that have been sitting out (because the bacteria builds up on the plates at room temperature).
- On a picnic, carry perishable foods in a cooler with a cold pack or ice and keep them in the shade.
- Keep hot food hot! Keep cold food cold!

Resources

FDA Consumer Information Line (800) 532-4440 or (301) 827-4420

FDA Seafood Hotline (800) FDA-4010 or (202) 205-4314

USDA's Meat and Poultry Hotline (800) 535-4555 or (202) 720-3333

Safe Tables Our Priority (STOP), a nonprofit grass roots organization focused on the issue of food poisoning, devoted to victim assistance, public education, and policy advocacy for safe food and public health. Hotline 800-350-STOP and information clearing house.

Web Sites:

National Food Safety Initiative:<http://vm.cfsan.fda.gov/>

FDA's Home Page: <www.fda.gov>

Centers for Disease Control—information on "bad bugs"<www.cdc.gov>

Also check with

Your local health department

Nontoxic pest control:

Whatever Works—offers many nontoxic and low-toxicity products for pest control Brooklyn, New York (800) 947-8374

Harmony—environmentally conscious products for the home, located in Bloomfield, CO (800) 456-1139

Books:

Deborah Lynn Dadd, *The Nontoxic Home & Office* (1992) and *Home, Safe Home* (1996) both Tarcher / Putnam Book, New York.

Ann Louise Gittleman, *Guess What Came to Dinner,* Avery Publishing Group, Inc., Garden City Park, New York, 1993

Amy Kyle, *Contaminated Catch: The Public Health Threat from Toxics in Fish*, National Resources Defense Council, Washington, DC, 1997

CHAPTER TEN

Food Storage and Recycling

◆

Another critical aspect of maintaining a safe and healthy kitchen is looking at both food storage and that critical modern appliance, the refrigerator, so important in keeping our food safe and fresh. It is vital to store foods properly in order to prevent spoilage and vulnerability to pests and to preserve the wholesomeness of food as long as possible. Environmental and health issues related to the containers in which our food is packaged is another concern. Even though plastics are a great invention, their ongoing production creates higher amounts of pollution. Food packaging affects the Earth's overall well-being, and doing our part to recycle can make a significant difference.

THE REFRIGERATOR

The refrigerator is the central "foodquarters" of most kitchens and offers protection against food spoilage and contamination. The key is to keep it organized and clean, and to use the food you buy in a timely manner. Assess your refrigerator shelves (and cupboards) on a regular basis and look for items that should be used before they spoil. It is helpful to organize your refrigerator into separate areas of food types, such as dairy products, breads and other grain products, vegetables, condiments, etc. This not only helps you find what you need quickly, it's also helpful when you are putting away your groceries or checking on what needs to be used first. I actually like to bag my groceries at the store, organizing them by where they will be stored away in my home. **Also, if I place all the refrigerator items in one bag, they keep each other cold and cozy on the way home.**

Keeping Track of What's in the Fridge

I enjoy going to the market and choosing the freshest produce of the day and creating a menu around my choices, rather than planning a meal and then shopping for the appropriate ingredients. I also like to investigate my refrigerator on a daily basis, pulling out what needs to be used and what "calls" to me; then I place those items on my counter and figure out my menu from these selections. This is one way to use the food we buy without waste. If I notice that there are vegetables that need to be used up, for example, I might make a soup to serve with whole grain bread, or make stir-fried vegetables over rice.

On the other hand, my wife Tara, who also cooks in the same kitchen, likes to keep her favorite foods at the front of the refrigerator shelves and use primarily those foods. If I don't rotate them, I might find some colorful relics at the back of our refrigerator. And then to the trash or recycling it goes, whatever it was. "Rotate and Rejuvenate" (place the new items behind the old to avoid foods going bad) was my father's slogan for stocking the shelves and produce counters at our family store, where I worked during my teen years.

Your Refrigerator and Cupboards Reflect Your Health

When I was a country doctor, embracing the new philosophy of the nutritional medicine movement, over twenty years ago, I often requested a home visit to new patients, especially those families with children. Besides the patient interview, I would ask for a tour of their kitchen so that I could look through their cupboards and refrigerator to assess their cleanliness and health habits and get a sense of their diet. Although some patients were uncomfortable with this, it was a mutually informative experience, shedding light on the relationship of diet to health. I might pull out items, ask questions, point out food additive concerns, and often make associations between dietary habits and my patients' health. For example, if the family was frequently ill with colds and flus, bronchitis and ear infections, I would often find milk products including cow's milk, cheese, and ice cream, along with many processed foods, such as breads, crackers, and cookies. In families with chronic illness, I often observed a notable absence of fresh fruits, vegetables, and whole grains. I spoke with my patients about bringing more nutritious and cleansing fruits and vegetables into the family diet, decreasing the congesting dairy products and sugary foods to support the outcomes of greater immune resistance, fewer infections, and reduced congestion.

Another common relationship between food and health is often seen in families who focus on meat and potatoes, with an emphasis on milk products and processed foods. These foods are also congestive and add to cardiovascular risk. I have seen the effects of such diets reflected in my patient's elevated blood pressures and cholesterol readings.

I found that involving the children in my early kitchen tours was often quite helpful. By enlisting their participation in improving the family diet the whole family got educated about healthy nutrition and shopping wisely.

Nowadays, there is much more awareness about the relationship of diet and health. However, parents still unwittingly contribute to their children's diet problems by setting a poor example themselves. *My number one guideline for feeding kids healthfully and establishing lifelong food habits is: set a good example!*

Parents are usually the ones who do the shopping and who make the choices that fill refrigerators and cupboards. And nothing a parent says will have as much impact on a child as what that parent does. So the earlier a healthy plan is implemented in the household, the sooner these positive habits can become part of a lifelong approach to good health.

Storing Perishables

- After shopping, unload perishables (items that need refrigeration, such as milk, eggs, etc.) and frozen foods first, and immediately refrigerate or freeze them.
- Store dried foods (such as grains and pasta) and root vegetables (such as potatoes and onions, that can also be refrigerated) in a closed pantry or other cool, dry area. Don't store them directly under a sink, and always keep foods off the floor and separate from chemicals and cleaning supplies.
- If you can, wash your fruits and vegetables thoroughly when you get them home (or do it before you prepare them), then refrigerate them at 40°F or below. Most fruits, such as apples or oranges, can be left at room temperature for many days, however, they will last longer when refrigerated.
- To make sure that you rid your fruits and vegetables of E. coli and other bacteria, soak them for 20 minutes in a solution with Organo-clean or another coconut oil-based soap designed as a vegetable wash.
- Keep fresh vegetables and fruits refrigerated in plastic bags.
- Keep other whole foods, such as grains and beans, in covered glass or plastic containers, out of direct light.

- Store eggs in their carton inside the refrigerator to keep them cold, rather than on the refrigerator door where it's warmer.
- Nuts and seeds stay freshest when stored in the refrigerator or freezer.
- Check the labels on condiments and other foods that need to be refrigerated once they're opened.
- Since animal proteins spoil the most easily of all foods, store securely wrapped packages of meat, poultry, or fish (that you intend to use in 1 to 2 days) in the meat drawer or coldest section of the fridge. Be sure that juices don't drip and contaminate other foods. Immediately freeze any fish, meat, or poultry that will not be cooked within 2 days. Lunchmeats can usually remain safely in the refrigerator for a week or two, or go by the labeled safety dates.
- When storing leftovers, divide foods into shallow containers for rapid cooling.
- Slice foods such as egg dishes into serving-size portions so the food will be thoroughly chilled.
- Use cooked leftovers within 4 days. If you want to be super organized, you can keep labels and a pen in the kitchen and date leftovers.
- Periodically, double-check the temperature of your refrigerator with an appliance thermometer. The temperature should be 40°F.

Frozen Food Guidelines

- You can freeze almost anything except canned foods and eggs in shells. Once food is out of the can, you can freeze it.
- Foods stored at 0°F are protected from the growth of microbes such as bacteria and molds, which enter a dormant state. However, once thawed, bacteria again become active, and can multiply rapidly. So after the food is thawed, cook it immediately and thoroughly to destroy any microbes.
- Check the temperature of your freezer or freezing compartment every so often, or keep a thermometer in it. The temperature needs to be 0°F or below to assure safe storage.
- The FDA reports that freezing does not destroy nutrient content. Freezing does slow enzyme activity, for better and for worse.
- Frozen cans can cause health problems. Never use foods frozen in a can.
- If there's a power failure, keep the refrigerator and freezer doors closed. Add blue

COLD FOOD STORAGE GUIDELINES

Product	Refrigerator, Unopened	Refrigerator, Opened	In Freezer
Casseroles, homemade		3-4 days	1-2 months
Homemade or deli salads: macaroni, egg, chicken, tuna		3-5 days	No
Pre-frozen casseroles TV dinners			3-4 months. Keep frozen until ready to eat
Vacuum-packed dinners	2 weeks	3-4 days	3-4 months
Soups and stews		3-4 days	2-3 months
Egg whites/egg substitutes	10 days	3 days opened	12 months
Fresh in shell	3-5 weeks		Do not freeze
Hard-boiled	1 week in shell	3 days	Do not freeze
Cooked egg dishes		2-3 days	
Milk	see dates	5-7 days	1 month
Swiss, brick, processed cheese	2-3 months/ date	3-4 weeks	Affects texture and taste
Chicken, Whole, uncooked		1-2 days	12 months
Cooked		3-4 days	4 months
Canned poultry	2-3 years	3-4 days	
Fish, Lean (such as cod)		1-2 days	Up to 6 months
Fatty (blues, perch, salmon)		1-2 days	2-3 months
Gravy		1-2 days	3 months
Hot dogs	2 weeks	1 week	1-2 months
Deli & lunch meat	2 weeks	3-5 days	Do not freeze well
Ground Beef		1-2 days	3-4 months
Steaks and Roasts		3-5 days	6-12 months
Pork Chops		3-5 days	3-4 months
Roasts, uncooked sausage		1-2 days	1-2 months

Source: Food and Drug Administration Web Site, <www.fda.gov>; from Food Marketing Institute for fish and dairy products, USDA for other foods.

ice or dry ice to keep things cold until the power returns. A separate free-standing chest or upright freezer will keep food frozen for 2 days if it's fully loaded.

- You can protect against loss of frozen food by freezing quarter-gallon jugs of spring water. This provides extra refrigerant, should the power go out, and also large amounts of bottled water in case of emergency. Or you can buy freezer gels (blue ice).

- Perishable items can be refrozen if they still contain ice crystals or feel cold to the touch.

- Discard any food that is room temperature. But don't taste it—food may look and smell fine, and yet contain dangerous bacteria. When in doubt, throw it out!

FOOD STORAGE

Foods can spoil. It's a simple fact. Most fresh fruits and vegetables, depending on their ripeness and refrigeration, must be used within a few days to a week or two at most. Leafy green vegetables usually need to be used within the week, while root vegetables may be stable for several weeks in the refrigerator. Fresh meats, poultry, and fish, which are most easily contaminated by bacteria, must be refrigerated and used within 2 days, or they should be frozen immediately. Dairy products must be refrigerated, and it is a good idea to keep an eye on the expiration dates. Taking a minute to smell your milk is a good habit to develop as well. Whole grains and beans store well (in dry cool areas) because of their protective coverings; when free of insecticides, they can be kept indefinitely, or at least a year or two. They should be kept in sealed containers to avoid insects. On the other hand, flours, which are ground grain, lose their protective coverings and should be kept in the refrigerator or freezer. Nuts and seeds are definitely best refrigerated or stored in the freezer, because they contain oils and easily become rancid.

The containers in which we store foods are important to their protection and longevity. Plastic containers with airtight lids have become very popular and appear to be safe for storing grains and grain products because they are lighter than glass, which is also a popular storage material. Sealed plastic bags (like the zip-lock type) are effective for items stored in the refrigerator. Since plastic bags are more susceptible to insects and mice, they should not be used for storage in the cupboard. Any container should prevent moisture from getting in, which can cause the food to break down. Foods that are prone to microbe contamination should be stored in the refrigerator.

Many foods that are prepackaged in boxes, cans, or jars contain some kind of spoilage retardants and do fairly well when stored in cupboards. However, opened packages of cereals, crackers, and other grain products should be closed securely and used within the month or refrigerated to protect them from insect infestation, especially during the warmer months, because the smell of grains will attract grain moths, mice, and other critters.

Other Storage Contaminants

- Some types of ceramics have lead in the glaze. Do not use any acidic foods, such as fruit juices or tomato sauce, in these ceramic containers.

- Avoid the use of antique or collectible housewares for food and beverages as they also can contain toxic metals.

- Do not store beverages in lead crystal containers, as this can add toxins.

- Avoid storing food in cabinets under the sink or near water, a drain, or heating pipes. Food can attract insects and rodents through the openings to the pipes.

- Select your pots and pans with care: stainless steel and glazed ironware appear to be the safest choices. Avoid aluminum and also copper cookware until the last word is in on their toxicity. In the case of aluminum, it has been linked with Alzheimer's disease in several studies.

Pantry Pests

Bugs! Mice! Pests! Interesting in nature, but not much fun in the kitchen. Some of the vermin that affect food include ants, grain moths, mice, rats, flies, cockroaches, and the germs carried by these insects.

Insects and other pests find their way in from the outside through cracks and crevices or on items carried into the house. Since infestations are most likely to occur in packages that have been opened and then left unsealed and unrefrigerated, it is helpful to store food in jars, tins, or other tightly sealed containers once they've been opened. A single package of food can become home to large numbers of insects. Ants are notorious for bringing their whole village over to dine on some crumbs or surround a jar of honey.

What to do? When a kitchen pest problem develops, our primary task is to find and remove the food or material that has been infested. Then examine all exposed food, including opened packages of cereals, dried fruits, nutmeats, flour, meal, corn-

DRY FOOD STORAGE GUIDELINES		
Food Item	**Storage Time**	**Specifics**
Canned fruits and vegetables	1 year, possibly more (unopened cans on the cupboard shelf)	After opening, remove from can and refrigerate
Chocolate, baking or powder	18 months	Keep in a cool cupboard
Coffee	1 to 2 years in can	Refrigerate or freeze Freezing keeps it freshest
Dry milk (nonfat)	6 months (unopened or sealed)	Keep airtight in fridge
Flour, unbleached Whole wheat flour	8 months to 1 year 3-6 months	Refrigerating is best Refrigerate whole wheat
Honey and maple syrup	1 year, unopened 6 mon. opened (maple in fridge)	Do not feed honey to young children
Mayonnaise and dressings	6-12 months	Keep in refrigerator no more than 3 months after opening
Molasses Oil, vegetable oil, olive	6-12 months 3 months after opening 12 months	Keep tightly covered Store in refrigerator Store in cool dark place

starch, crackers, breakfast foods, dehydrated foods, macaroni, chocolate, cocoa, dry soup mixes, spices of all kinds, dry dog food, and birdseed. Many kinds of insects have become highly adapted to feeding on stored flour, bran, and other processed grain products. All sources of infestation need to be found and eliminated. **If there is any doubt as to whether or not a food is infested, it should be discarded.** If you suspect insects in a packaged food but they can't be seen, you can also put the packages in sealed plastic bags for a few days and monitor them for bugs. Any food that seems to be vulnerable to insect attack should be purchased only in small quantities and stored in the refrigerator.

Once insects have had the opportunity to make themselves at home throughout the kitchen, it is essential to remove all the pantry contents, clean the shelves, and use a nontoxic product to discourage them. Fortunately, there are a number of excellent nontoxic solutions to insect problems on the market, many of them based on borax or boric acid. (See Resources for Whatever Works, Pest Control Products)

Food Item	Storage Time	Specifics
Pasta—macaroni egg noodles	1-2 years 6 months	Keep airtight
Peanut butter	Refrigerate after opening 6-9 months	Can turn rancid when exposed to air or heat
Rice, white *Rice, brown*	1-2 years 1-2 years	Keep in airtight containers
Salad dressings	6-12 months Refrigerate after opening	Keep in refrigerator
Spices, whole ground herbs	1-2 years 6 months	Heat and long-term storage can reduce color and aroma
Nuts and seeds, raw	3-6 months	In refrigerator or freezer
Nuts, sealed vacuum packed	1 year or see date	In cupboard

Source: Adapted from Iowa State University and Kansas State University in the *Mayo Clinic Health Letter*, October 1996.
Note: For most items, opened is not that different from unopened if item is sealed securely. Anything that could become rancid, such as whole grains or nuts and seeds, will do best stored in the refrigerator.

Remember that your refrigerator is one of your best protections against pests. In fact, this is another good reason to refrigerate all perishables immediately. However, when cold-storing grain or grain products, note that molds can also be a problem and can attract insects as well, so keep flours tightly sealed, even when in the refrigerator, to protect them from moisture.

A Few Tips for Preventing Pests from Living In or Around Your House

- Take away their food supply by keeping living areas clean. Be especially careful to sweep up food crumbs, wipe up spills when they happen, wash dishes immediately, and deposit leftover food in its proper place. Store food in tightly closed, impenetrable metal, glass, or hard plastic containers. Empty garbage cans frequently and, if necessary, accumulate garbage in a plastic bag with a twist tie to eliminate the enticing odors of decaying food.

- Dry up their water supply. Repair leaky faucets, pipes, and clogged drains. Insects have to drink somewhere—don't let poor plumbing turn your home into the "neighborhood bug bar."

- Get rid of any clutter that they can hide in. [The rest is basically off the topic of food and kitchen storage.] Clean out your attic, basement, and closets. Remove piles of old clothing, newspapers and magazines, and boxes. Check out-of-the-way places (under stairwells, for instance) where unused items often get tossed.

Survival Preparation: Food Storage

An important question to ask yourself and family or housemates is, "Are we set up to survive 1 week if we are cut off from resources and supplies?" Any number of natural disasters and human catastrophes—earthquakes, floods, fires, road damage, etc.—could affect our water, electricity, phone, TV (Oh, NO!), or the road to our home. Even in the city, we should have at least three days worth of water and food supplies on hand.

Such supplies should be storable for at least a year. You should also check your supplies every 6 months or so and use or replace whatever needs updating. You'll need at least 2 quarts of water for each person per day. If you have a large pantry, you could store more. Canned goods store well, and packets of dried soups (made by adding hot water) are nourishing foods and lighter for storage. Also, important and potentially vital foods include dried beans and seeds, which can be used to sprout nutritious foods in a few days.

If you want to have canned soups and other canned foods, you may need a small stove with propane gas, or you could use your barbecue if you maintain a sufficient supply of propane or charcoal. Obviously, perishable foods should be used first. After that, use dried foods or anything else with a shorter storage life than canned goods.

Our local utility company offered a great tip in one of their newsletters. They suggested freezing quarts or liters of drinking water, as many as you have room for. These blocks of ice can then help keep food cold for awhile if the power goes out and your refrigerator isn't working. As these bottles melt, you'll also have good water to drink. Also, smaller frozen plastic water bottles can be used to keep picnics and lunches cold and provide cold drinking water as well.

Food for emergency supplies should be stored in a protected place, such as a cool dark storeroom. I know people who bury emergency food in large sealed containers, where the ground is at a relatively consistent temperature. In general, we want our survival food and supplies safe and readily available, should we need it.

COMMON PESTS OF STORED FOOD

Pest	Concerns	Attractions	Solutions
Ants	Invasive pest; some species bite or sting; some can carry disease	Sweet, fatty, and protein foods (sugared foods, grain products, such as crackers and cookies, peanut butter, meats, etc.); water.	Destroy outside nest; various chemical ant traps; natural treatments—sprinkle red chili pepper, paprika, dried peppermint, or borax; plant mint around the house
Beetles	Allergic reactions from breathing fragments; intestinal distress, irritation, and possible infection from ingesting larvae	Grains, cereals, other grain products, dried fruits, sweets, spices; some species infest meat, fish, cheese; cat and dog food	Good hygiene; use tight-fitting #30 mesh screens on doors; check packaged foods before you bring them home; store food in containers; avoid moldy foods; cook meats thoroughly
Cockroaches	Transmission of disease—commonly salmonella, toxoplasmosis, and others; allergies	Bags, cartons, any human or animal food; water; can live inside TVs, alarm clocks, radios, love answering machines, and even refrigerators!	Good housekeeping: no food out overnight; use boric acid; "The Meal" and electronic roach zapper (Whatever Works); jar traps (see Dadd)
Flies	May transmit diarrhea, typhoid, cholera, polio, intestinal worms, eye infection, salmonella, shigella	All foods; garbage, lawn clippings, any kind of decaying matter	Remove garbage promptly; use tight-fitting screens; eliminate food sources; hang clusters of cloves; citrus oil aromatherapy; flypaper
Mites	Dermatitis, respiratory allergies	Products high in fat: peanuts, cheese, ham; sweets; grains	Refrigerate foods; use sealed containers
Moths	Avoid ingesting larvae	Flour, cereal, biscuits, nuts, dried fruit, chocolate, dog food	Replace staples frequently; store in closed containers; refrigerate flours; discard any "webby" food; sift flours (#64 mesh)
Rodents: rats and mice	Can carry insects and disease, such as viruses and the germ that causes plague	Attracted to food, garbage, may infest walls of homes	Get a cat; use mouse traps baited with peanut butter; nontoxic repellents and traps (Whatever Works)

Sources: Debra Dadd. *The Nontoxic Home & Office* (Putnam, 1992)
Walter Ebeling. *Urban Entomology* (out of print, but available on the Internet) <http://cnas.vcr.edu/~ento/>
Whatever Works, Pest Control Products, Brooklyn, NY (800) 947-8374

RECYCLING

Recycling is a crucial concept and practice for the well-being of our planet. With all the people and all the production in our world at this time, we need to be extremely conscious of environmental resources and those activities which affect them. One of the key questions to ask in regard to our personal consumption is: where did this product come from and where is it going? In other words, by using this particular product, how am I enhancing or depleting the Earth's resources?

The idea of conserving the Earth's resources underlies the basic philosophy of this book: purchase and consume, as much as possible, foods grown from local organic farmers or from your own garden, yard, or deck. Fresh fruits, vegetables, whole grains, beans, nuts, and seeds have their own inherent natural recycling— they come from the Earth and any unused portions can go back into the Earth without causing any damage. If we compost our food wastes and use them in our garden or window boxes, this is the essence, the very definition of recycling. When we buy local, natural products, we are conserving gasoline used in transportation, as well as the wastes generated to process foods and create packaging.

In buying used and recycled products, we are saving the costs (to the environment) of making something anew. By sharing tools and other products with neighbors, we are conserving resources. We can also shop more conscientiously with regard to the containers in which our foods or products come. Recyclable containers include glass bottles and jars, aluminum and other metal cans, cardboard, papers, and even some plastics.

We all know instinctively that recycling is good for the environment and therefore good for us. But did you know that it's also good for business? In 1994 for example, 565 million pounds of plastic containers made of polyethylene-terephthalate (PET) were recycled. At prices of 10 to 40¢ a pound, that's a return of $56 million dollars or more.

Similarly, glass bottles are being recycled in greater numbers. Wine bottles can be washed and reused, which has been standard practice in Europe for many years. A vineyard can collect and wash a bottle for 40% of the cost of a new bottle. Refillable milk bottles are also making a comeback and are reported to save consumers somewhere between 4 and 12¢ on the half gallon. Glass milk containers are refilled on average 20 to 30 times before they're broken or lost. And plastic milk jugs (made from high-density polyethylene or polycarbonate resin) are typically refilled 50

RECYCLING IS IMPORTANT BECAUSE:

- The average American produces about 4 pounds of garbage daily.
- Americans go through 2.5 million plastic bottles every hour.
- We throw away enough glass bottles and jars to fill the 1,350-foot twin towers of New York's Trade Center every two weeks.
- We throw away enough iron and steel every day to supply all the nation's automakers' daily needs.
- Individual and industrial consumers in the United States throw away enough aluminum to rebuild our entire commercial air fleet every three months.
- Recycled paper requires 60% less energy and 15% less water. One ton of recycled paper saves: 17 trees, 7000 gallons of water, 4200 kilowatts of energy, 3 cubic yards of landfill.
- Packaging costs about 10% of total product cost.
- Twenty-five million tons of acid rain are generated each year from sulfur dioxide and nitrogen oxides spewed from factories.

Source: from *Staying Healthy with Nutrition* (see page 486).
Sources are Environmental Defense Fund and *Save Our Planet.* (Dell, 1990)

---

times before being discarded, according to industry sources. Also, plastic bottles can be melted to remake other plastic goods.

There are many other meaningful ways to recycle which you can build into your kitchen routines. If you have access to a recycling center, consider having 3 or 4 containers in the kitchen, pantry, or laundry room—for glass, cans, plastics, and paper. Glossy magazine paper is also recyclable. When shopping, try to buy fewer goods that need recycling; this moves you to more wholesome, fresh products which should be the basics of a healthy diet, and will help minimize the necessity for recycling in your household.

Suggestions for Reducing Waste and Avoiding Toxic Products

- Avoid Chlorofluorocarbon (CFC) products, such as polystyrene (Styrofoam) containers and packaging protectors, whose production and breakdown are polluting the atmosphere and destroying the ozone layer.

- Avoid aerosol sprays, such as deodorants, hairsprays, cleaners, and paints.

RECYCLING

What can you recycle or buy recycled, including foods, containers, and other items used at home?

Newspapers, which account for millions of trees annually

Aluminum beverage cans—about 50% comes from used cans that were melted to make new

Glass bottles and jars, including beer, milk, soft drinks, & wine bottles—nearly 25% of the glass in bottles and jars has been used before

Plastic bottles and jugs: for juice, water, and milk

Tin cans—tin cans are actually made of steel, about 25% of which is recycled steel

Cardboard egg cartons, fruit trays, and flower pots are made of recycled paper

Phone books and other paper, including glossy magazines

Paperboard boxes for cereal, crackers, etc.

Paper towels and paper napkins

Toilet paper and facial tissue

Shopping bags, or use your own bag of paper or cloth

Use rental equipment whenever possible instead of purchasing it

Donate or recycle large and small appliances; buy rebuilt or used equipment

Put crumbled toast and seeds in the bird feeder

Use vegetable scraps to compost for the garden or window boxes

- Reduce your use of plastic wrappings and containers, or use products with comparably minimal waste, for example bulk cheese instead of individually wrapped slices.
- Use biodegradable products, such as paper (instead of plastic); water-based soaps; eggs packed in cardboard; waxed paper rather than plastic wrap.
- Purchase reusable products, such as cloth napkins and towels, returnable bottles, and rechargable batteries.
- Recycle everything possible, such as glass, cans, paper, cardboard, plastics.
- Reuse as much as possible, such as paper bags, plastic bags, cardboard boxes, bottles, Styrofoam packing pellets, rubber bands, office supplies.

- Buy more durable products.
- Buy less of everything whenever possible.
- Shop at co-ops and farmer's markets where products are available in bulk. There are less fancy and costly packaging, and they support using recycled plastic and paper bags.
- Buy in bulk or get larger containers in place of six-packs, or large containers of regularly used products, such as soaps, detergents, shampoos, and cleansers.
- Voice your objections to stores and manufacturers when you spot new throw-away, nonrecyclable products; the plastic can and the throw-away camera are two recent examples.
- Ask your supermarket to stock more biodegradable products.
- Support legislation for deposits on bottles, cans, and plastic containers.
- Borrow or rent items that you only need infrequently, and keep other items in good repair; loan them to neighbors, also. (Make responsible agreements for shared maintenance and repairs if you do.)
- Minimize the purchase of plastics, styrofoam, and other nonbiodegradable products. Precycling means not buying products you cannot recycle. This will create a demand for the production of environmentally sound packaging.
- Packaging information laws are slowly changing to help consumers learn more about what they are buying. If you choose to purchase packaged foods, try to make conscientious, healthy, and environmentally sound choices.

Resources

For questions about the safety of a specific food: FDA Consumer Hotline (301) 443-1240

The Green Kitchen Handbook, Annie Berthold-Bond and Mothers & Others for a Livable Planet, HarperPerennial, New York, 1997.

Guide to Buying Recycled Products for Consumers and Small Business (1996) Pennsylvania Resources Council, PO Box 88, Media PA 19063

Real Goods Catalogue of Earth conscious materials (800) 749-0252 <www.realgoods.com>.

Seventh Generation for recycled paper products (800) 456-1191 <recycle@seventhgen.com>.

Alpine Aire specialize in freeze-dried, shelf-stable foods (800) 266-7777 <www.btt.org>

Environmental Defense Fund (800) 684-3322 <www.edf.org>

Whatever Works, Pest Control Products, Brooklyn, NY (800) 947-8374

CHAPTER ELEVEN

Eating Healthy Away from Home

◆

Generally, the best way to insure a safe and healthy diet is to eat meals prepared in your own home, ideally from the freshest and most wholesome ingredients. However, many of us are eating away from home more than ever before. We have busy work schedules and busy lives, and to save time we often grab ready-made food and eat on the run. Some people may even eat the majority of their meals in restaurants. But government data shows that we are twice as likely to become sick after eating out. Between 1983 and 1992, 42% of all reported food-poisoning outbreaks were traced to food eaten in restaurants, delis, or cafeterias. Only 21% of the cases of food poisoning were attributed to food eaten at home.

When you travel or go out to eat, unless you are going to a very health conscious restaurant or someone else's home whom you can trust to prepare healthy meals, what's on the menu may not only be high in chemicals, fats, sugars, and salt, it may also be germ-contaminated due to unhealthy food handling practices. Check the restrooms before you order a meal. I have found that a dirty restroom is a pretty good indication of an unsanitary kitchen. So, just as we need to be cautious when we make our selections in the market, eating out requires that we take certain steps to insure our health.

Here are five basic guidelines for eating out and staying healthy:

- Preparing and eating the majority of your meals at home gives you and your family the greatest control over your diet. This is better for your budget and your health.

- Save dining out as a treat, and when you do, make healthy choices.

- If you work long hours, develop a repertoire of wholesome, tasty bagged lunches and dinners to bring with you.

- Try to assess the cleanliness of the restaurant before you decide to dine there. There may be times when your observations and intuition save you considerable discomfort and unnecessary medical bills.

- Carry nutritional supplements with you to aid digestion and protect your health.

Protecting Yourself When Eating Out

There are a variety of foods and supplements that can offer protection against indigestion or possible exposures to microbes when eating out or traveling. Certain foods that may help support the digestive tract and nourish the stomach can be consumed in small amounts before going out or can be used during travel. If you are going to have a drink or two before you eat, there are several oils that will coat the stomach and slow the absorption of alcohol. Sometimes I eat a few pieces of kim chee, a tasty Korean dish of spiced cabbage, before I go out to eat—as a way to support my digestive process.

DIGESTIVE PROTECTION WHEN EATING OUT

Protective Foods	Protective Supplements
Cabbage	Ginger capsules
Essential oils, such as omega-3 fatty acids	Cayenne pepper capsules
	Garlic capsules
Olive oil	Vitamin C (typically 1,000 mg caps)
Kim chee—Korean spiced cabbage	Vitamin E (typically 400 IUs)
Nuts or seeds, a small handful	Digestive enzymes & betaine hydrochloride

With regard to supplements, I usually take 1,000 mg of vitamin C and 400 IUs of vitamin E before I go out to dinner. In addition, I put a few digestive enzymes in my pocket to take right after I eat, as well as one or two capsules of betaine hydrochloride to take with protein foods.

There is also a tendency to eat more than usual or to combine too many foods when you're eating out or at a party. Inappropriate food combinations (too many different foods or eating sugars with proteins, for example) and overeating can lead to a variety of complaints—from simply "feeling stuffed," to uncomfortable gas and bloating, to abdominal and back pains from the increased pressure in the intestinal tract. So the simplest advice is to eat as moderately as you can.

EATING HEALTHY WHILE TRAVELING

When I am traveling by air and staying in hotels, I usually pack some compact, nourishing foods such as almonds and sunflower seeds, healthy protein bars, a couple of organic apples, and at least a quart or more of purified or spring water. I also bring a variety of herbs and nutritional supplements, such as antioxidant nutrients, to deal with travel stress and chemical exposures. These include vitamins C and E, selenium, and beta-carotene, or an antioxidant formula that may include even more protectors and immune supporters, such as glutathione, L-cysteine, and lipoic acid. In addition, I'll pack digestive supplements like enzymes, hydrochloric acid (HCl), and probiotics, i.e., healthy bacteria.

DR. ELSON'S NUTRITIONAL TRAVEL KIT

Purified or spring water
Nutrition bars (protein-based energy bars)
Snacks: apples, nuts, seeds
Packets of miso broth

Packets of Emergen-C (powdered vitamin C with extra B-vitamins and minerals)
Herbal tea bags (my favorites)

Supplements: Vitamins C, E, and A
Antioxidant formula

Digestive enzymes and Betaine HCl
Probiotics (L. acidophilus and other healthy bacteria)
Aloe vera caps and other specific herbs
Immune supporters like echinacea and goldenseal
Blue-green algae tablets or capsules

When traveling to areas where food and water contamination is a concern, supplements are a must. Microbes do not populate and grow well in acidic environments or with stronger competitive microorganisms; therefore, taking HCl and probiotics can offer protection from food poisoning. Also, I drink only purified or bottled water, peel all fruits, and try to stick to cooked foods.

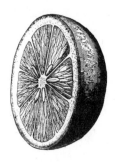

Six Tips on Staying Well When Traveling Abroad

- Boil or filter all water to "absolute 1 micron" or finer before drinking.

- Drink only beverages made with boiled water, canned or carbonated bottled drinks, beer, or wine.

- Make sure ice is made from boiled water only, or avoid it.

- Eat only cooked food, served while still hot. Avoid uncooked vegetables and salads.

- Eat only fruits that can be peeled.

- Avoid all raw foods including unpasteurized milk and cheeses, raw meat, seafood, and shellfish.

When traveling and selecting restaurants, it can be helpful to get advice and referrals from local people. If you have particular concerns about certain types of foods, such as vegetarian, low-fat, or low-salt, or if you just need a place you can be assured is conscientious and clean, read a restaurant review or check with the hotel staff for guidance. Look in the phone book under Health Foods and Restaurants.

It is also helpful to purchase simple snacks you can eat in your hotel room, such as water and lemons (for lemon water), other fruit, bagels, nuts, or cheeses (if you have a little fridge), for example. This reduces the number of meals eaten out and your room service bill.

RESTAURANTS

It is wise to limit the number of meals we eat out because of the many hidden ingredients, such as sugar, fats, excessive salt, and chemical additives, as well as exposure to other people's germs. Also, there is a tendency to eat more than usual and to have less discretion about the amount of calories and fats we consume, especially when eating at buffet-style restaurants or fast-food establishments.

For example, most baked goods and sauces used in restaurants are high in calories from sugars and fats, unless they are labeled differently on the menu or unless you really know how the chef is preparing the food. Professional food preparation techniques are not usually oriented to lower-fat or lower-sodium dishes. Frying and deep-frying using lower-quality oils are common, as is cutting costs by using less expensive ingredients or buying more preserved foods in larger quantities. I usually ask the wait staff, who are sometimes unaware of how the food is actually prepared, very specific questions about what ingredients are used, and whether any healthful alternatives are available within their restaurant.

We must be particularly cautious when choosing where we eat away from home. A survey of 45 state and local government agencies found that only 13% were enforcing the FDA Food Code cooking temperatures for pork, eggs, fish, and poultry! And only 64% required hamburgers to be cooked to 155°F, the minimum temperature necessary to destroy E. coli 0157:H7. (Center for Science in the Public Interest, 1996)

Do whatever you can to make sure that you choose a restaurant that is clean and appealing and that the foods used are fresh. If you can see the chef, make sure that he or she and the staff look clean and healthy. When the food is served, smell it and taste it first before gobbling it down. Be aware of heavily salty tastes and ask whether such additives as MSG or sulfites are used. For example, more Chinese restaurants now advertise that they use no MSG, or will at least avoid using it in your food if you ask.

Since restaurants are in business to turn a profit, they often attempt to cut costs with cheaper ingredients, bulk items, and processed foods that are less likely to spoil. They may not be buying the best or most wholesome fruits, vegetables, or other ingredients, and it is unlikely that they are purchasing organic produce. However, there are exceptions throughout the country, as organically oriented restaurants continue to open and thrive.

I believe that anyone who charges money for food should be painstakingly careful in purchasing, storing, and preparing the foods they serve; however, that is not always the case, which is why there is an increased risk of becoming ill when you eat out. The cleanliness of the restaurant and the health of the food preparers and servers should be a top priority. How do they clean their cooking utensils and, more importantly, your eating utensils? Are their sponges and cutting boards clean? Are the owners aware of their worker's health conditions, and do they have clear guidelines for when they can and cannot handle food in the restaurant? Do they use chemicals to which you might be sensitive? If it doesn't appear that they are attentive to cleanliness issues such as these, you may wish to dine elsewhere.

In any situation in life, we are usually presented with positive and negative choices. Restaurants are no exception. The following brief reviews of popular cuisines will suggest foods to regard with caution or to consider as occasional treats, as well as those that represent a healthier choice. I will also point out the dominant flavors of each style of cooking. Of course, most restaurants offer all flavors—sweet, salty, spicy, sour, and bitter. However, many of us focus primarily on two or three, particularly sweet and salty foods. For a balanced diet, seek out a variety of flavors over the course of the day whenever possible.

Restaurant Specialties

American

Flavors: Sweet, salty, and a creamy texture.

Concerns or Occasional Treats: Deep-fried and fatty foods, using low-quality vegetable oils and hydrogenated fats; refined flour and sugar products; fatty meats and potatoes, like burgers and fries or meatloaf and gravy; iceberg lettuce salads with lots of dressing; cheese sauces; macaroni and cheese; chicken and potato salads, heavy with mayonnaise; pot pies, which are high in salt, calories, and saturated fats; dishes made with butter or heavy cream; along with high-fat and high-calorie shakes, ice cream, and rich desserts of cakes or pies.

(*The lower quality American menu, such as hamburgers, fries, and shakes, is probably the riskiest of all the cuisines listed here. A regular diet of such foods tends to lead to the common degenerative diseases, including cancer, heart conditions, and diabetes.*)

Healthier Choices: There is a healthier version of American cuisine now served in most cities, often referred to as "California" or "Nouvelle" cuisine. Pastas and fresh vegetables, grain and bean dishes, lower-fat soups and sauces, and fresh fish are usually featured. California cuisine is similar to a Mediterranean diet, which emphasizes the freshest foods in season and creating the menu from those. A glass of wine or bottled mineral water is often the beverage of choice. The new, reasonably priced rotisserie turkey and chicken restaurants, with lots of vegetable side dishes, are healthier choices. Choose the white meat; baked or sautéed potatoes rather than mashed (which often have added cream and butter); rice; fresh salads; steamed or seasoned vegetables; sweet corn; and other entrees without cheeses.

Fast American Foods

Flavors: Salty, sweet, and greasy.

Cautions: We want it now! This apparently perfect solution to our fast-paced, working society is not that at all. This low-cost food may save time, but it is usually very high in fats, sugars, salt, and refined ingredients. It is often comprised of fried meats, high-fat fries, sugary sodas, and shakes, and should be considered an occasional treat (like once a month).

Healthier Choices: Not many, although some fast food establishments may offer a veggie burger, grilled chicken sandwich, or a salad. Look for stuffed pita pockets and a variety of "wraps" now being featured. Order your sandwiches without the mayo. And opt for fat-free or low-cal dressing for the salad, or ask for lemon wedges and skip the dressing.

Mexican

Flavors: Spicy, salty.

Concerns or Occasional Treats: Products with animal fats, refried beans with lard; fried chips and any fried foods; excess cheese and sour cream; and excess salt in most everything.

Healthier Choices: In many Mexican restaurants you can order low-fat refried beans without added lard. Other good choices include vegetarian burritos; whole grain tortillas; lightly oiled chips; fresh salsa without additives; guacamole without added mayonnaise; non-fried chicken or fish in the tacos, burritos, or other menu items. Go easy on the chips and enjoy the salsa, tostadas, and other vegetable-oriented dishes.

Mexican Fast Foods

Flavors: Salty, spicy, and greasy.

Concerns or Occasional Treats: This may be even worse than the standard Mexican fare with higher fats and oils, lard in the beans, salt, and lower quality meats.

Healthier Choices: You may be able to purchase vegetarian burritos made with vegetable oils rather than lard, with lettuce and tomato. There are also veggie or chicken fajitas, non-fried items, and even low-fat items in some Mexican fast food outlets.

Italian

Flavors: Spicy, sweet.

Concerns or Occasional Treats: The Italians really want to see you enjoy your meal, so watch the temptation to overeat because of the great flavors and generous portions. Don't eat too much bread and butter, heavy cream sauces, preserved meats, and heavily salted foods. The dishes highest in fats include fettucini Alfredo and breaded or fried dishes such as breaded veal and fried calamari.

Healthier Choices: There are many good choices in most Italian restaurants: pastas in a variety of light, meat-free sauces, such as tomato or garlic and olive oil; fresh or grilled vegetables; minestrone and pasta soups; fresh fish and baked chicken; and salads. Also, a glass of wine, or better yet, sparkling mineral water can be a refreshing beverage.

Chinese

Flavors: Sweet, sour, salty, and sometimes spicy.

Concerns and Occasional Treats: Dishes that are very sweet, such as sweet and sour sauces; fatty foods, such as breaded or batter-dipped foods like crispy beef or pork dishes; deep-fried or fried foods like egg rolls, fried noodles, and fried rice. Assume MSG is included unless the menu specifically says it is not. Be cautious of excess salt and oils, and sometimes lower-quality fried meats and poultry.

Healthier Choices: Most Chinese restaurants also offer healthy fare—lightly sautéed vegetables with rice and modest amounts of meat, fish, poultry, or tofu; and no added MSG. Szechuan dishes with hot peppers, hot sauces, or mustards can be stimulating if you enjoy spices. Minimize added salt and soy sauce.

Japanese

Flavors: Salty, spicy, bitter.

Concerns and Occasional Treats: Deep-fried tempura; raw fish (due to the potential contamination of the fish by parasites or bacteria in the raw fish); too much salt from the soy sauce; sweeteners in the sauces; and food coloring in the spicy horseradish (wasabi). If you have high blood pressure, go easy on the soy sauce.

Healthier Choices: Japanese food has interesting flavors and is light, yet filling. Good selections include vegetable sushis, tofu dishes, cooked seafood dishes, noodles and soups, and seaweed, which is very nutritious.

Thai

Flavors: Sweet, spicy.

Concerns and Occasional Treats: Sweet sauces; rich coconut sauces and soups, which contain more saturated fats; and go light on the peanut sauce, which can be quite caloric.

Healthier Choices: Thai restaurants usually offer tasty low-fat sauces and healthy entrees. As with most Asian foods, they are best when they provide the right balance of fresh vegetables along with rice and a small amount of protein, be it meat, fish, poultry, or tofu.

French

Flavors: Subtle flavors, creamy and smooth textures.

Concerns or Occasional Treats: Buttery and cream-based sauces, high in fats and calories; bread and butter; cream soups; specialty sausages; heavy desserts, also high in calories and fats.

Healthier Choices: Here in the States, there has been a trend in recent years to lower the fat and cream used in French restaurants. Fresh fish and lightly buttered vegetables, good salads with light vinaigrette dressings, and lighter desserts are healthy, but still tasty French restaurant selections.

Middle Eastern

Flavors: Salty, bitter.

Concerns or Occasional Treats: Watch for the high oil content of fried foods, such as falafels and heavy meat dishes. However, in general this is relatively healthy fare.

Healthier Choices: There are a lot of light dishes to try: tabouli (couscous with tomatoes and parsley); hummus; babaganouj (eggplant dip); pita breads; salads; and olives.

BUFFETS AND POT LUCKS

The all-you-can-eat buffets are one of the biggest food challenges. How much and how many different foods can your stomach hold and still function safely? How do huge meals affect your health? And how will you feel the next day? Unfortunately, our body doesn't function like a snake's, so we can't eat one huge meal and then eat nothing for days. Still, if you do tend to overeat at a party or pot luck—and I have done that a few too many times in my life—you can limit your food intake beforehand and afterwards.

It takes strategy to eat a healthy meal at a buffet restaurant or pot luck party. Avoiding excesses is the key to avoid feeling stuffed and uncomfortable. Limit your choices to six or seven, including desserts. Try to choose simply made dishes, and limit yourself to only a few tastes of fattening or rich foods. Also, limit your intake of artificial-looking concoctions. For example, choose some green salad, a rice or pasta dish, some vegetables, and focus on 1 (or a maximum of 2) entrees, and 1 (maybe 2) desserts (a taste or two of each is better).

When you are cooking for a pot luck, make something wholesome that you enjoy and know you can eat. Then you'll have a safe choice for yourself that you can also share with others. (Does your offering tell them something about your personality? Are you sweet and gooey, crunchy and flavorful, or meaty and hardy?) And for those of you who are overweight or challenged by allergies or other health issues, try to follow your personal guidelines for foods to avoid.

Another factor at the buffet table is hygiene. Hopefully, you are eating with people who share your values about cleanliness and follow basic hygienic guidelines. Each bowl or pot should have its own serving utensil, and everyone should use the servers and not their personal silverware. And no double dipping! Do not put food back into the bowl after you have already taken a bite.

Before I eat a big meal or go to a party, I drink a glass or two of water and some vitamin C-nutrient powder like Emergen-C, or I take 1,000 mg of C with bioflavonoids and about 400 to 800 IUs of vitamin E. I also bring some digestive enzymes and acidophilus/probiotics (healthy bacteria). If the evening is going to be long and my energy is low, I might take blue-green algae and sublingual vitamin B-drops.

DR. ELSON'S GOING-TO-A-PARTY PLAN

1. Before the Meal—Before you go out or at least half an hour before you eat:
   Drink 1 to 2 glasses of water with: Vitamin C powder (like Emergen-C) or 1,000 mg of C with bioflavonoids and 400-800 IUs vitamin E
2. Bring Along with You—to take with or right after the meal: Digestive enzymes and acidophilus/probiotics
3. If It's Going to Be a Long Night, and Your Energy is Low—also take before you go out: Blue-green algae and sublingual vitamin B drops (high in B_{12})

EATING ON AIRPLANES

Since we are exposed to so many stressors when we fly—poor air quality, dehydration, germ exposure, a variety of chemicals, extended sitting and inactivity—we want to avoid further stress from consuming the wrong foods and drinks. We need to take extra special care of our bodies when we travel. In particular, we should avoid excessively salty foods and alcohol, which contribute to dehydration and can lead to sinus problems, constipation, swollen legs, and low energy.

I usually order vegetarian meals when I fly, and that way I at least avoid processed animal protein, which put extra stress on the body. Special airline meals need to be ordered when you make your travel reservations.

I also travel with snacks, a healthy sandwich, and water, just in case my special meal doesn't meet my needs. This is even more important for longer trips, as are all these concerns and cautions. Other wholesome travel snacks include: fresh fruit, nuts and seeds (almonds, walnuts, sunflower seeds, and pumpkin seeds), trail mix (nuts, seeds, and raisins), protein energy bars, and whatever else you like that's healthy and travels safely. Remember that eating perishable foods that are kept too long at room temperature is the greatest single cause of food poisoning. You can also buy healthy carry-out meals or snacks in many airports.

DR. ELSON'S AIRPLANE PLAN

- Taking vitamins and additional antioxidants, including vitamins C and E, selenium, and zinc, as well as some extra minerals, to prevent the ill effects of germ exposure and stress.

- Drinking water before, during, and after your flight to prevent the adverse effects of dehydration and constipation.

- Packets of powdered vitamin C and Bs (or liquid Bs), plus minerals (such as Emergen-C by Alacer) to improve hydration and protect cells and tissues from the stress and radiation exposure of travel.

- Aloe vera capsules or other laxative, cleansing herbs to keep the digestive tract moving—one or two caps at bedtime are helpful. It is a good idea to try your choice of cleansing herbs before you travel so you can predict their effects.

- Relaxation or sleep herbs, or melatonin for sleep when crossing time zones.

- After you land, drink plenty of water and make sure you sleep well.

VENDING MACHINES

Vending machines used to offer only processed and preserved food, such as sodas, candy bars, cookies, and crackers. These contain a lot of sugar, calories, fats, food coloring, and salt. Nowadays, we can often find healthier snacks in vending machines, including juices, waters, sandwiches, and whole grain muffins. However, these still may not be totally wholesome, so we shouldn't count on vending machines for anything other than emergency snacks.

One of the keys to healthy eating is to plan your meals and snacks *before* you get hungry. Bring your own good quality food to work or school so that you have what you need when you need it. If you can't make your own meals and snacks, find out where to go to get good, healthy food in your neighborhood and near your job.

HOSPITAL FOOD

Wouldn't it be nice if our hospitals served their patients food that looked and tasted like it would generate healing? Unfortunately, hospital food is like any other institutional food—made in large quantities with many refined and processed ingredients and plenty of additives. Of course, there are all kinds of special diets that doctors order for their patients, such as bland, low-salt, low-sugar, and low-fat diets, or diets with a specific sodium or calorie count. Other than these specifications, however, the fundamental healthfulness of hospital meals is not a strong consideration. Yet, when we are ill, we need the most healing diet possible, and I take that to mean fresh, vital, and wholesome foods—fresh juices, soups and salads, fresh steamed vegetables, light and nourishing proteins, fresh fruits, and other supportive nourishment.

So, if you or a loved one needs to spend time in a hospital, bring in nourishing food that is appropriate to their medical needs. This usually includes fresh fruit or vegetable juices, soups, salads, and freshly made food with which the patient is familiar.

In following any specific dietary regime, be it wheat- or dairy-free, high-protein, low-carbohydrate, vegetarian, or whatever, it is helpful to create guidelines and customize some menu plans. Have food available to your family when it is time to eat. *This usually means thinking ahead and creating meals and snacks before you leave home.* If this isn't possible, be sure you know where you can go to get what is on your plan. When you are not prepared, at work for example, and it's 2 PM and you still haven't eaten, your food discrimination level may be diminished and you will likely veer from your dietary path. And what is typically available in your local store or restaurant is precisely what you may be trying to avoid. So, bringing good food, even leftovers, to work or school, is the best and often most economical and healthiest choice you have.

CHAPTER TWELVE

Nourishing Our Children

♦

I know that it's difficult to change your habits for the benefit of others; this needs to be something you do for yourself. However, if anyone should make positive changes, it is parents for the sake of their children.

Here are my top-ten guidelines for parents who want to teach their children good nutritional habits.

Guideline Number One: The most effective way to get kids to eat healthfully is to **set a good example!** Young people are most influenced by what they see and experience, not by what they're told. Therefore, what you do—how you live—has the greatest effect on shaping your kids' behavior and their diets. Remember that the habits your children form while they're young will probably be with them for life.

Begin your good example by assessing your own eating habits and buying wholesome foods for your family. Avoid habits that you know are destructive, especially in front of your children. Don't smoke (ever), drink alcohol, drink excessive coffee, or consume junk foods—other than on special occasions. Most of these unhealthy habits are likely to be picked up by your young ones. Why not have them "inherit" healthy habits instead?

Guideline Number Two: Feed your children a balanced diet. Natural tastes for food develop early. If kids eat real food and develop a taste for fruits, vegetables, and other delicious flavors from Nature, they won't depend on the "enhanced" flavor of processed food. Continue to cultivate their tastes for natural foods, even after they have experienced the intensely sweet flavor of chocolate cake, sodas, and ice cream, or the highly salty flavor of chips and pretzels. Make sure your kids eat a nutritional meal first before allowing treats or desserts.

A balanced diet for you and your children includes 70 to 80% wholesome, natural foods—whole grains, legumes, fruits and vegetables, nuts and seeds (if well tolerated), quality dairy products, and animal proteins (if these are desired). Limit treats and watch out for excess sugar, caffeine in sodas and chocolates, and heavily processed foods laced with chemicals like colored dyes and preservatives.

An important part of a balanced diet also involves getting plenty of fluids—good drinking water should be a basic for everyone. Children may need to be encouraged to drink water before having other liquids, especially sugary drinks. Consider getting a filter or buying bottled water so that you can make good tasting and healthy drinking water available for the entire family.

Guideline Number Three: Don't bribe your kids with sugar and other treats; encourage them with healthy foods and snacks. It is so easy to forget to take the time to deal with children's true needs—which are love and attention. When you're busy, it's tempting to give them sodas, sweets, or whatever, even TV, instead of you. This can create the habit of trying to satisfy emotional needs with the distraction of food or material things. If your child adopts this pattern, it can lead to a lifetime of sugar abuse and obesity and all of the problems that result from the misplaced attempt to satisfy a basic human need.

Guideline Number Four: Have healthy snacks around the house for your kids— organic sliced apples, oranges, grapes or bananas; raisins or dates; almonds or other nuts; yogurt; pieces of cheese with healthy crackers; good chips and guacamole or salsa; and more. Offer your children healthy snacks at least a couple of times a day, such as mid-morning or in their school lunch, and then after school, around 3 to 4 PM (a time some parents call the witching hour—recognizing that their kids are becoming cranky and irritable, but not realizing that they may simply be fatigued or have low blood sugar).

Guideline Number Five: Get your children (over age 5) involved in shopping for and preparing the foods that they like. When you go to the grocery store, allow them to choose a few appropriate treats. You could give them a budget, maybe $10, to spend on good choices when they help you shop for family groceries. Most children will appreciate learning to prepare food that they like. Younger ones will be enthused about playing "kitchen" and "restaurant" with siblings or parents. Typically, kids enjoy making smoothies and shakes, preparing pasta and sauce, arranging fruit or veggies on a platter in a pretty design. When age-appropriate, help them learn to cut up fruits and vegetables or snack foods and prepare basic recipes. Fruit salads are often a big hit. And be creative; together you may find some new taste treats.

Guideline Number Six: Plant a garden with your kids if you have the space, or if not, join with neighbors in a community garden. If you have only a patio or small deck, you can use planter boxes or hydroponic equipment to cultivate organic, quick-growing produce. Even if you only have a window sill, there are many food-producing plants that will fit in a small space—tomatoes, strawberries, herbs, and lettuce, for example. It is magical for kids to watch things grow and eat foods fresh off the vine. My daughter loves to pick and eat strawberries, raspberries, sweet peas, cherry tomatoes, and fresh sweet corn out of our garden. Or get your kids to help you make tasty, nourishing, and vital sprouts from seeds or beans, such as alfalfa, sunflower, lentils, or mung beans.

Guideline Number Seven: Organize your refrigerator and pantries in a way that allows the young ones to get the items that you want them to have. This makes it harder for them to get to the treats that you want to control. Even if they eat too much junk when they're with their friends or at school, encourage them to eat well when they're home, and keep setting a good example. It will be worth it for you too in the long run!

Guideline Number Eight: Help your children to avoid or to limit their intake of foods with unhealthy additives. (You can review this issue more thoroughly in Chapter 4.) The basic additives to watch out for with regard to children are: artificial food colors, excess refined sugar, MSG (monosodium glutamate), aspartame (an artificial sweetener), sodium nitrite in treated meats, excess sulfites in dried fruits and other preserved foods, hydrogenated fats, and the new Olestra. I also limit my children's intake of foods containing artificial flavorings, the preservatives BHT and BHA, and excess salt.

Guideline Number Nine: Look out for food allergies and reactions that are so common in children. (They may manifest in ways that are not typically thought to be food related, even by some physicians, but it is vitally important to address possible allergies.) You will notice that when children limit foods causing their reactions, they will usually become clearer, more alert, and healthier. A delayed food allergy can cause a "hidden" reaction that may not appear until later that day or the next. For example, chronic ear fluid congestion (otitis media) is quite common in young children. This is often not an infection, but is usually treated as though it were, with strong antibiotics. When children who have chronic ear infections are taken off cow's milk products, those with a dairy allergy or sensitivity will stop getting ear problems.

FOODS AND ADDITIVES TO AVOID TO KEEP KIDS HEALTHY

Additives To Be Cautious About

Additives	Source
Sugar	Many foods—check the label for "sugars"
Aspartame & Saccharin	Diet sodas, baked goods
Artificial Colorings	Drinks, candies, cakes, confections
Sulfites	Dried fruits
MSG (Monosodium Glutamate)	Chinese food, canned soups (check the label)
Caffeine	Some sodas, chocolate
Nitrites and Nitrates	Hot dogs, lunch meats
BHA, BHT	Some perishable foods, crackers and cereals

Food Treats and Related Health Concerns

Additives	Source
Nonorganic Strawberries	Highest in pesticides of any fruit
Sodas & Colored Drinks	Aspartame, sugar, artificial food coloring
Fried Foods	Deep fried fats linked to heart conditions
Fast Foods	High levels of fats and sugars
Candy	Sugar, fats, and artificial colors

Other problems related to allergies include skin problems, mood swings, and certain digestive complaints. Some of the most common foods that cause allergic or allergy-like reactions in kids, besides milk are: eggs, peanuts, citrus fruits, and tomatoes. Since any food can cause an allergic reaction in any individual at any age, it is wise for parents and their doctor to pay attention to this possibility.

A Word about Cow's Milk: This is a controversial subject for anyone who isn't in the dairy industry. Cow's milk is a double-edged sword; its nutritional value is tempered by allergy, fat, and cholesterol risks. Cow's milk is for baby cows and not for humans. Although some children and adults handle it fine, milk contains complex proteins that are difficult for young children to handle, and it can set up an allergic reaction and lead to a general allergic state. I have always been concerned about the effects of the homogenization process and the high heat of pasteurization on our body and blood fats. At our house, we didn't give either of our children cow's milk in their first few years; instead we used more soy milk and some goat's milk, which are less allergenic.

Guideline Number Ten: Consider giving your children protective nutrient supplements. Common nutritional deficiencies in children include iron, zinc, calcium, vitamins A and C, plus a variety of B vitamins. Just as kids can get too much of a food or an additive, they can also unknowingly be getting too little of a particular nutrient. The nutrient needs of younger children are much greater than the needs of adolescents and adults. A newborn infant needs about 60 calories for every pound of body weight, whereas an adult needs only about 12 to 18 calories. So

HEALTHY ALTERNATIVES TO NOT-SO-HEALTHY KID FOODS

Typical Choices	Healthier Choices
Soda	Juice drinks, water, natural sodas
Hamburgers	Lean turkey or beef burgers, vegetarian burgers
Hot dogs	Chicken or turkey dogs (nitrite-free), tofu or vegetarian dogs
Bologna	Nitrite-free chicken or turkey, veggie bologna
Whole milk	Skim or 1% milk, organic when possible, soy milk or rice milk
Processed cheese	Wholesome cheeses without food coloring
French fries	Baked fries or baked potatoes
Pizza loaded with cheese and meat	Pizza with less cheese and more veggies, burritos and wraps
Candy bars	Fruits, almonds, protein bars
Cookies	Whole wheat animal, fruit juice sweetened whole grain cookies, fig bars, or graham crackers
Milkshakes	Home-made fruit smoothies
Ice cream	Ice cream without additives, frozen or fresh organic strawberries, peaches, or raspberries, watermelon, oranges, cantaloupe in season

without adequate nutrition, children can become malnourished much more quickly. Children don't need a lot of additional vitamins and minerals, especially if they are on a healthy, balanced diet. However, the requirement for many nutrients is high during the growing years, and providing nutritional insurance by giving your children a few additional supplements over and above their diet is a good idea. I suggest an age-appropriate multi-vitamin and mineral combination, preferably one from natural sources and without preservatives, sugar, or artificial food coloring. There are a variety of healthy brands at natural foods stores and available through catalogs, and even pharmacies have good choices. Additional vitamin C, in amounts of 100 to 250 mg twice a day, is usually helpful. Even more can be given if the child has allergies or becomes ill with a viral problem like a cold or flu. When kids are under stress, exercising more, traveling on airplanes, or when they are exposed to chemicals, an antioxidant may be protective; look for one that contains vitamins E and C, beta-carotene, a little selenium, and zinc. I like the chewable Oxy-Bears from Douglas Lab in Pittsburgh. Also, children really enjoy the Emergen-C powdered products from Alacer Corporation; about a half packet (500 mg) is appropriate for most children over age 4. These are another good way to supply additional vitamin C and trace minerals.

HEALTHY SNACKS

Whole Wheat Toast	Organic Fresh Fruits:
Organic Tortillas, Corn or Wheat	Apples, Pears, Peaches
Refried Beans	Grapes, Bananas, etc.
Brown Rice	Raisins and other Dried Fruits
Rice Cakes	Fruit Smoothies
Cookies, whole grain with fruit juice sweetener	Almonds
Oatmeal, with milk or yogurt	Sunflower Seeds
Little green salads	Hearts of romaine with dressing
Carrots	Baked Potato
Celery, especially the tender inner stalks	Chicken
Black Olives	Tuna
Organic Peanut or Almond Butter	Yogurt

RECIPES KIDS LIKE

Family Burritos

Ingredients: Whole wheat or corn tortillas, refried beans, brown rice, black olives, cheddar or jack cheese, mild salsa, and chopped lettuce. Options: corn off the cob, sliced avocado or guacamole, or chopped tomatoes.

I first make a pot of brown rice by boiling 4 cups of water with a couple pinches of sea salt and 1 to 2 teaspoons of olive oil added just before the 2 cups of brown rice. Turn down the heat and lightly simmer in the covered pot. (The rice is optional because the tortillas can serve as the grain.)

My thirteen-year-old son opens the cans of organic refried beans and black olives while my eight-year-old daughter grates a small pile of cheese. (Parents can judge appropriate jobs for their children.) My wife chops the lettuce and slices a tomato, and I heat the skillet and get my tortillas lined up. I also mash the bean mixture in a small bowl and mix in a little of our favorite salsa; then I heat it a minute in the microwave, which helps the filling stay warm and melt the cheese. You can even mix in the rice and cut olives into the beans, and then have one substance to place in the tortillas, especially if you have young children who can only handle one ingredient. Be sure it's not too hot to touch.

I place a few drops of oil in the medium hot skillet and heat one side of the tortilla to light brown; then I flip it and let the other side brown while we put in the filling, sprinkle cheese on it, and fold it. This allows double the time to brown both halves of the second side of the tortilla, which you'll need to flip one more time. Then we put the burritos on a plate, open them slightly to put in whatever else we each want—salsa, olives, lettuce, tomato, even leftover salad, and then put a splash of our favorite salad dressing on the burrito if we want to. One or two of these family burritos is a full meal!

Fruit Juice Popsicles

These are so easy to make, economical and tasty! Take your favorite fruit juices, organic if possible, and pour them into ice cube trays or in popsicle makers with the appropriate sticks. Some good choices include orange juice, apple juice, juice blends, pineapple coconut, and grape. Avoid artificial food colorings and use the healthiest and freshest juices possible.

Chicken, Vegetables, and Baked Fries

Take your favorite parts of chicken—ideally from free-range or organic birds—and place them in a covered ceramic cooking dish. Chop some onion and garlic for flavoring, carrots, potatoes, and whatever other veggies (which become extra flavorful) the kids like. Put a few tablespoons of water in the dish and season all the ingredients with butter or a light olive oil basting, salt or soy sauce, garlic powder or other seasonings, such as pepper, rosemary, and other favorites.

Bake in the oven at 350°F for 30 to 45 minutes until done. Serve with rice or with home-baked fries.

Home-Baked Fries

Cut 4 or 5 whole baking potatoes (with skins) lengthwise into the right size for fries. Drip some olive oil onto your clean hands and lightly rub the potatoes, or toss with a little olive oil in a bowl. Place them on a baking sheet and sprinkle with sea salt or other seasoning. Bake them for 20 to 30 minutes in the oven at 350°F.

Vegetable Soup

Start with a soup pot and add a quart or two of water. Heat on a medium setting. Let the children choose from the vegetables you have preselected: onions, carrots, potatoes, cauliflower, green or purple cabbage, zucchini. Chop the vegetables and place those that need to cook longer in the pot first. Begin a slow simmer for 10 to 15 minutes. Then have the children add the other vegetables. Also, have them open a can of stewed tomatoes or tomato sauce. Add any of the following spices to taste: salt, garlic or onion powder, pepper, and others your family likes. I also use a good quality vegetable/protein soup-base powder that I buy in the health food store and add some toward the end of simmering. I may also have the children open a can or two of vegetable or minestrone soup, or chicken soup or broth, and add that to bring more flavor and for thickening. You can also extend your soup with some rice or pasta, giving it a heartier flavor and making it a more substantial meal. Serve with your favorite healthy bread or crackers that are low in hydrogenated fats, sugar, and additives.

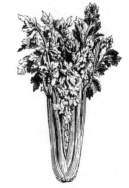

A Few Words about School Cafeterias

The typical school cafeteria generally offers meals with too much refined flour and sugars, starch, excess cheese, and artificial food colorings. Also, fast-food conglomerates are beginning to buy their way into many school cafeterias across the country. I am sorry, but I cannot accept as a balanced meal for our children a high-fat cheeseburger, French fries, and a sugary soda or a milkshake. Nor is processed macaroni and cheese and chocolate cake my idea of good nutrition. I ate these kinds of meals growing up and was fat and congested with colds and allergies. I rarely give this sort of stuff to my children and they are trim and healthy.

Although I've heard that such healthy items as fresh fruits and vegetables are being offered at some schools, and while food awareness and nutrition are improving in this country, the reality is that many unhealthy food choices are still being offered to our children.

The USDA oversees school lunch programs, and they seem to be supportive of the food industry giants. Much of the free food supplied by the government to schools is on my "avoid" list—hydrogenated vegetable oils, orange-colored cheeses, peanut butter with added hydrogenated fats and sugar, refined white breads with additives, and other processed food.

The food service people are not necessarily to blame. They have limited funds, many regulations, and little support from the government to change. So, they say "give the kids what they like to eat," because they need to sell meals to keep afloat. When they try to make some improvements, they often end up combining healthy ideas with poor ingredients. For example, one school began to make oatmeal for 50 to 100 kids, but with 3 pounds of sugar and 5 pounds of margarine (straight hydrogenated fats). "But that's the only way the kids will eat it," they claimed. Some schools in Hawaii began to bake their own bread, an admirable undertaking; yet, their primary ingredients were refined flour, margarine, sugar, and dried milk. Even potentially healthier vegetarian nachos include chips with plenty of fried hydrogenated fats and processed cheese with food coloring.

The most common excuse is that kids won't eat anything else. And that may be true if the food is similar to, or even better than, the diet they get at home. Still, school lunches should be nourishing and healthy. Otherwise, the kids may be hyped up or dopey on sugar and food chemicals, which is hardly ideal for learning or cooperative behavior.

Parents must be encouraged to become involved in their local school's lunch program and in their own children's diet. In some schools, where health-oriented food and cooking classes are available, there is greater acceptance of more wholesome snacks and meals.

If you want to make sure your kids get the nourishment they need, send a wholesome, balanced bag-lunch to school with them!

WHAT TO PACK IN A HEALTHY SCHOOL LUNCH

Note: Have a good lunchbox or one of the new thermal bags that keeps food hot or cold.

- Sandwiches—on nutritious whole grain bread:
  Tuna salad
  Turkey (oven-roasted or other nitrite-free packaged or deli turkey)
  Almond or other nut butter with a natural fruit jam (conserve) or sliced banana and honey
- Apple or slices in a small sealed container
- Other sliced fruit or a whole orange or banana
- Raisins (organic and sulfite-free if possible)
- Almonds or other nuts or seeds in a small baggie or container
- Sliced carrots or celery
- Leftovers from last night's dinner (baked chicken, burritos or enchiladas, pasta, etc.)
- Juice and water mixture, or just water, in a small thermos, or a chilled plastic bottle of water to keep lunch cool

Resource

My book, *Staying Healthy With Nutrition*, has a number of relevant sections on nutrition for children, including Chapter 15's individual Lifestyle Programs on *Infants*, *Children* and *Adolescents*, as is appropriate for your family. Chapter 14 includes a variety of recipes especially for children.

Ten Ways to Encourage Children's Healthy Eating Habits

1. Set a good example by eating a healthy diet yourself.

2. Provide a balanced diet with a variety of tasty and nutritious foods.

3. Avoid using food as a reward and encourage healthy snacks.

4. Have healthy snacks available, and offer them to your children at appropriate times, such as mid-morning when they're home and in the afternoon after school.

5. Get kids involved in shopping and cooking.

6. Help children grow fresh food in a garden or planter box.

7. Organize your refrigerator and cupboards so that kids can get the right stuff for them.

8. Avoid the riskiest food additives—artificial colors, aspartame, BHT, MSG, and excess sugar.

9. Look out for allergies and food reactions.

10. Ask your health practitioner about a quality children's multi-vitamin/mineral (without additives and artificial colorings), as well as a little extra vitamin C, calcium, or any other appropriate children's supplement.

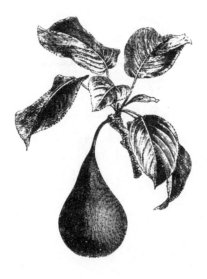

IN SUMMARY

There are obviously many areas of importance for conscientious shopping, eating a healthy diet, and creating a health-supporting lifestyle to protect our well-being and prevent diseases over our lifetime. Eating a wholesome and balanced diet, getting regular exercise and proper sleep, managing stress, and keeping a positive attitude toward life (which leads us to treat ourselves in ways respectful to our body) are some of the basics of healthy living. Avoiding abuses of food and substances is also crucial to our long-term health.

10 MOST IMPORTANT IDEAS FOR SHOPPING AND STAYING HEALTHY

1. Have your diet include as much wholesome, fresh food as possible.

2. Buy and consume as much of your food as possible organically grown.

3. It is important that the foods you and your family eat regularly be organic to avoid accumulated toxins.

4. When possible, buy your foods in season and from your locale, as these are usually more economical and less toxic.

5. Limit your intake of processed foods.

6. Specifically, avoid nitrites, sulfites, MSG, Olestra, and artificial colors.

7. Avoid excessive or regular intake of SNACCs— Sugar, Nicotine, Alcohol, Caffeine, and Chemicals (from foods and drugs).

8. Don't overeat, but do chew your food well and take time to eat.

9. Drink noncontaminated water as your primary beverage in amounts appropriate for your needs.

10. Set a good example for yourself and your family by maintaining and creating healthy eating habits.

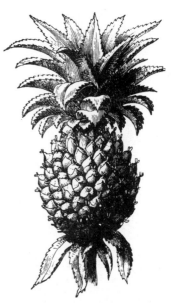

APPENDIX
Common Food Additives

Of the more than 3,000 different chemicals that are used in preparing foods for sale to consumers, only some are true "food additives"—agents actually added to the foods and listed on the ingredient label. Many of these are GRAS (Generally Recognized as Safe) list additives. There are also many unlisted chemicals that include solvents such as formaldehyde, benzene, and carbon tetrachloride—all carcinogens used to extract salad oils—that may contaminate our food. The body of this text discusses many of these concerns. The best we can do is to be aware of what is known and demand that the government and food growers give us complete information.

This appendix offers you support to Chapters 5 and 6 of this book in exploring food labels and individual food additives. NOTE: For each of the following food additives, I have provided you with a simple rating from one to four stars (*). I have limited the four-star additives because the overall goal for a healthy diet is to limit processed foods and thus, food additives. This appendix will help you to become more "chemically intelligent."

*	Avoid
**	Use only occasionally
***	Use in moderation
****	Okay to use regularly

Common Individual Food Additives

***Acacia / gum arabic** (GRAS)—A complex sugar originally extracted from the acacia tree. Soluble in water and in foods, it retards sugar crystallization, and acts as a thickener and blending agent. Used in the confection industry for candies, jellies and glazes, and chewing gum, and as a stabilizer in soft drinks and beer. Gum arabic is safe according to most studies.

*Ace-K / acesulfame potassium**—The most recently developed artificial sweetener now being added to beverages and diet foods. Found to cause tumors in animals. Avoid. (See Chapter 4 for more.)

***Acetic acid / sodium acetate / sodium diacetate** (GRAS)—The acid in vinegar, it is also found naturally in fruits, coffee, and wine. Used as an acidic flavoring agent for catsup, pickles, mayonnaise, wine, and some cheeses; found in any foods that are preserved in vinegar; also used as a synthetic flavoring agent (as ethyl acetate) in many beverages, processed cheeses, pickles, and processed foods. Considered a safe additive.

***Agar-agar / seaweed extract** (GRAS)—A tasteless polysaccharide made from several varieties of red algae. In liquid, it tends to thicken and gel, making it a good substitute for gelatin from animal proteins. Used in making ice creams, jellies, icings, preserves, and for thickening milk and cream. Agar also acts as a mild laxative and can be an allergen. It is used both by the food industry and sold in stores for home use. Agar-agar is a safe, even beneficial, food additive.

***Alginates: alginic acid; algin gum; sodium and other mineral alginates** (GRAS)—These natural extracts of various seaweeds are used primarily as thickening and stabilizing agents to prevent ice crystal formation in foods such as ice cream, to distribute flavors in desserts, and to add smoothness to mixtures as in ice creams, custards, confections, and cheese spreads. All of these alginates are safe.

***Aluminum salts: alum (aluminum potassium sulfate); sodium aluminum phosphate; aluminum ammonium sulfate; aluminum calcium silicate; aluminum hydroxide; and others** (GRAS)—There have been concerns about accumulation of aluminum in the body and its effect on brain chemistry and health, particularly its relationship to Alzheimer's. Aluminum compounds are used to decrease acidity (as a buffer), as an astringent, to keep canned produce firm, to lighten food texture, and as anti-caking agents. Alum is used as a clarifier. Sodium aluminum phosphate, the most commonly used, is found in baking powder and self-rising flours. There are aluminum-free baking powders available, and substitutes for other aluminum products. Aluminum calcium silicate is used as an anticaking agent in salt; aluminum hydroxide is safe in small amounts used as a leavening agent in baked goods; and aluminum ammonium sulfate is used as a buffer and neutralizing agent by the cereal industry. In small amounts most of these aluminum salts seem to be well tolerated in food, but none should be used regularly. More research will guide us to know whether it should be avoided completely.

***Ammonium salts: ammonium bicarbonate; ammonium chloride; ammonium phosphate; ammonium sulfate** (GRAS)—Ammonium salts may occur naturally in foods. As an additive, used in foods as leavening agents for baked goods, and as dough conditioners and buffers to lighten texture, to create uniformity within a food mixture and to enhance flavor. With the exception of ammonium chloride, which can cause nausea, these salts have no known toxicity.

***Annatto** (GRAS)—A natural coloring agent extracted from the seeds of a tropical tree, Bixa orellano. It is a yellow/orange vegetable dye frequently used in dairy products such as butter and cheese. Also used to color margarine, ice cream, baked goods, and the casings of hot dogs. Annatto has no known toxicity.

****Ascorbic acid / vitamin C/ascorbate salts, as in calcium or sodium ascorbate, ascorbyl palmitate** (GRAS)—In both natural and synthetic forms, a beneficial vitamin essential for tissues, collagen, and blood vessels. Naturally found in many fruits and vegetables and used in food processing as an antioxidant and preservative to prevent oxidation and rancidity in fats and can preserve flavor, color, and aroma of the foods. Used as a nutritive additive for artificial fruit drinks and now in curing meats to prevent the formation of carcinogenic nitrosamines from nitrites. Nontoxic even in high amounts.

*Aspartame**—As the number one artificial sweetener, it has been with us as the tabletop Equal since 1980. A mixture of two amino acids, aspartic acid and phenylalanine, it is 200 times sweeter than sugar. As Nutrasweet, it is used in candies, diet foods, soft drinks, and chewing gums. People with PKU lack the enzyme to metabolize phenylalanine contained in aspartame, and may experience headache, dizziness, sleeping problems, and behavioral changes. Aspartame is an excitotoxin to the brain and should not be used by pregnant women or children as it could affect brain development. Research also linked aspartame to brain damage and brain tumors in animals. I do not recommend any regular use of aspartame.

Benzoic acid / *sodium benzoate (benzoate of sodium)* (GRAS)—Naturally occurring in berries and herbs, it is used as a preservative in a wide variety of processed foods, including margarine, soft drinks, juices, pickles, and condiments. Used as a flavoring agent in candies, beverages, baked goods, ice cream, and chewing gums. Probably the safest of the chemical preservatives. Larger amounts can cause intestinal upset, especially with weakened liver function, and there are allergies to these chemicals. Overall, small amounts of sodium benzoate seem to be safe.

BHA / *butylated hydroxyanisole* (GRAS) BHA and BHT are both petroleum by-products used as a preservative and antioxidant to prevent the rancidity of fats and spoilage that causes a change in taste, odor, or appearance. BHA is used commonly in many packaged and processed foods, such as dry cereals, crackers, instant potatoes, soups, canned or bottled beverages, shortening, baked goods, and more. Allergies to BHA have been known and liver toxicity is possible. There is further concern with carcinogenesis in Japanese rat studies and my advice is to avoid any regular use of the chemical BHA.

BHT—butylated hydroxytoluene (GRAS)—BHT (also see BHA) is a preservative used in processed foods such as enriched rice, breakfast cereals, shortenings, dog and cat foods, and cake mixes. BHT can be irritating to the liver and kidneys, especially when there is decreased function of these organs. Allergic reactions have also been known. There is also some concern that BHT may convert to other substances in the human body that may be carcinogenic. The use of BHT is prohibited in England. I suggest avoiding foods with BHT.

Caffeine (GRAS)—Found naturally in coffee, chocolate, tea, guarana root, and kola nuts. As part of coffee, tea, and cola (it's not on the label), it is one of the world's big drugs. Caffeine is a stimulant to the heart, brain, and lungs, and gives people "energy." Used as an ingredient in most cola and root beer. Caffeine use is only questionably safe, but it can cross the placental barrier, so it can affect the growing fetus and therefore, it is not recommended during pregnancy or during nursing. Children should avoid caffeine in drinks and chocolate, as should anyone with cardiovascular disease or ulcer problems. Regular use should clearly be avoided. (See the Caffeine chapter in *The Detox Diet*.)

***Calcium proprionate* / *proprionic acid/sodium pro-prionate* (GRAS)—Naturally found in dairy products such as butter and cheese, and used to prevent growth of fungi and bacteria; used as mold inhibitors in baked goods; and as preservatives in cheeses, chocolate products, and preserves. All are considered safe.

***Calcium salts:** calcium carbonate, chloride, citrate, gluconate, hydroxide, lactate, oxide, phosphate, and sulfate* (GRAS)—Helpful in providing calcium, an essential mineral, especially for healthy bones. Used in enriched foods, especially grain products and infant formulas; as emulsifiers in evaporated milk and frozen desserts; as dough conditioners in baked goods; clarifying agents in sweets; as a buffer in baking powder; and as firming agents in jellies or in canned produce. Their use in foods is considered safe.

Caramel—Made by heating sugar, giving it a burnt, slightly bittersweet taste. Used as a coloring for soft drinks such as colas and root beer, candies, ice cream, and baked goods—and in many different flavorings, such as butterscotch and ginger ale. There is some question about the safety of caramel. The heating process uses ammonia, which may be toxic, and other potentially harmful compounds. In modest doses, caramel is still considered safe.

***Carob, or locust bean gum* (GRAS)—An extract from the bean pods of the carob tree, it is a natural flavoring used as a healthier substitute for chocolate and sugar, as well as a flavoring for beverages, ice cream, candies, baked goods, and desserts. Used as a thickener and stabilizer in chocolate milk, syrups, desserts, and cheeses. Some recent concern, although not proven, for its safety in pregnant women. More likely, locust bean gum may be beneficial and lower cholesterol. Overall, considered safe.

****Carotene* / *beta-carotene* / *provitamin A* (GRAS)—Found naturally in many yellow/orange vegetables and fruits, such as carrots, sweet potatoes, and apricots. Converted to vitamin A in the body, it is a useful natural coloring agent in butter, margarine, and cheese. Also, a useful additive and helpful antioxidant. It is a safe additive, even in high dosages, where its only side effect is yellowish pigmentation of the skin.

***Carrageenan* / *Irish moss extract* (GRAS)—A gluey and salty seaweed extract used as a natural stabilizer and emulsifier in food processing, in such foods as French dressings, ice cream, sherbet, cheese products, and desserts. Thought to be safe, although there has been some concern about its effect on reproductive function and as an irritant in IBS, Irritable Bowel Syndrome.

Caseinates: *sodium, potassium, calcium, and ammonium* (GRAS)—As one of two major proteins in cow's milk (lactalbumin is the other), it is used as a texturizer in ice cream, ice milk, sherbet, and frozen custard. A nutritive protein source in many "protein" powders, binders or extenders in some lunchmeats and soups. Casein is essentially nontoxic. However, people who are allergic to milk or milk protein should avoid foods with added casein or caseinates.

Cellulose Derivatives: *carboxymethylcellulose, cellulose gum, methyl cellulose, and others* (GRAS)—The basic structure of plant tissues used in food processing as a thickener or stabilizer and emulssifier to blend ingredients and prevent caking in desserts such as ice cream. The cellulose derivatives are accepted as safe with no known toxicity.

***Citric acid and its salts:** *calcium, potassium, and sodium citrate* (GRAS)—Found naturally in fruits and commercially extracted from citrus fruit or made by fermenting crude sugar, it is used as a flavoring agent or enhancer to impart a tangy, tart, or sour taste to foods, including beverages, candy, ice cream, baked goods, and chewing gum. Used as a buffer to maintain acidity in foods such as fruit juices, carbonated beverages, wines, jellies, and sherbet. A firming agent in canned tomatoes and a vehicle for adding various mineral nutrients. Safe food additives.

Cornstarch—Mainly used to coat foods or containers to prevent sticking and as a thickener. Basically a safe additive, but not always listed on the label. It may cause mild allergic or intestinal symptoms in people sensitive to corn.

Corn Sweeteners: *corn syrup, high fructose corn syrup and corn sugar* (GRAS)—Corn syrup, the most commonly used corn sweetener, is made by chemically splitting cornstarch with a weak acid. Corn sweeteners are prevalent in the food industry as flavoring in various beverages, candies, baked products, ice cream, catsup, dressings, and many other foods. They are on the GRAS list with no limitations, and they seem to be safe overall, although they are caloric sugars that contribute to tooth decay and obesity if overused, as well as the ups and downs of sugar use. Occasional allergic reactions may also occur.

Cyclamate / Sucaryl—The cyclamates (sodium and calcium) were the diet sweeteners of the 1960s. When research showed that high amounts of cyclamates caused bladder cancer in lab animals, they were removed from the food market by the FDA in 1969.

Dextran (GRAS)—A polysaccharide produced by growing bacteria on sugar; it is used as a a foam stabilizer in beer and a mild sweetener as a substitute for barley malt. There is some concern about its safety, but it is still on the GRAS list.

Dextrin / starch gum (GRAS)—Dextrins are carbohydrates prepared by heating starches, such as cornstarch, potato starch, or tapioca. Used in food processing as a thickener in many sauces and gravies and as an expander in bakery goods. Dextrin is considered safe, and is basically metabolized easily as starch is in the body.

Dextrose—A form of glucose used as a sweetener in many beverages and packaged foods. It can be extracted from corn, sugar cane, or sugar beets, and like all sugars, its use should be minimized or avoided.

EDTA / ethylenediaminetetraacetic acid / calcium disodium (GRAS)—A mineral chelator that binds metals. Used more commonly as a preservative in salad dressings, mayonnaise, condiments, margarines, juices, and

drinks. EDTA tends to prevent changes in the color or flavor of foods. EDTA can cause kidney damage. Research on lab animals was inconclusive, but a link to cancer is possible. Being studied for toxicity.

Flavorings, Artificial—Literally thousands of chemicals are used to flavor foods. Minimize these additives and the foods that contain them. (See Chapter 4 for more information.)

Food Colors, Artificial—Not listed speficially on the label, other than Yellow #5 (tartrazine). However, they represent definite concerns. The following table briefly decribes the currently used artificial food colors.

Synthetic Colors in Current Use

• Citrus Red #2—Used in coloring oranges. Banned in 1976 from any other uses because it was shown to cause cancer in animals. It is important to avoid eating the rinds of oranges that contain this food coloring.
• Red #3 (erythrosine)—Used in cherries, gelatins, ice cream, fruit cocktail, candy, pudding, cereals, and baked goods. On the safe list, but is linked to possible genetic mutations, cancers, or changes in brain chemistry.
• Red #40 (Allura Red AC)—Took the place of banned Red #2 and is used in foods, drugs, and cosmetics. It may cause cancer in animals.
• Blue #1—A coal-tar derivative used in soft drinks, thirst quenchers, candy, ice cream, cereals, and puddings. A possible allergen, and it caused tumors in animals at the site of injection.
• Blue #2—Used like Blue #1 and is on the FDA safe list. The World Health Organization, however, has placed it in category B—questionable for use in food.
• Green #3—Used for green foods such as mint jelly, gelatins, candy, frozen desserts, and cereals. A potential allergen that caused tumors upon injection.
• Yellow #5 (tartrazine)—The most questionable color agent because it causes immediate allergic reactions in people sensitive to salicylates (aspirin). Asthmatics also tend to be allergic to yellow #5 more than the general population. By law, it is the only artificial color that must be listed by name on packaging. Tartrazine is used in yellow-colored foods such as spaghetti, puddings, gelatin, soft drink, sherbets, ice cream, cereals, and candy. Attempts to ban it have not succeeded. Most people can tolerate some Yellow #5 in foods, but those with sensitivity may develop skin reactions or asthma symptoms (problems are worse in sensitive asthmatics).
• Yellow #6—Another coal-tar color used in many foods, such as candies, baked goods, carbonated beverages, and gelatins. It is considered safe but linked to allergies.

Fructose—A natural sugar found in many fruits and in honey. Twice as sweet as sucrose, or cane sugar, fructose is used in candies, preserves, ice cream, and "natural" beverage drinks and ices. The health food industry often uses fructose instead of sucrose. It stimulates blood sugar and pancreatic insulin less rapidly than glucose (part of sucrose) and is absorbed more slowly. Fructose is basically safe in small amounts, as are most of the simple sugars. It is best to use fructose and other sugars moderately and to consume more natural fruits and vegetables to obtain the simple carbohydrates.

***Gelatin** (GRAS)—A tasteless and odorless protein made from collagen, animal connective tissue extracted from hooves, skin, snouts, tendons, or ligaments. Used as a thickener or stabilizer, and as a base in gelatin desserts, pudding, chocolate milk, whipped cream, and marsh-mallows, as well as in ice cream, sherbet, custard, and cheeses. Basically safe. Strict vegetarians usually avoid gelatin because of its animal origin.

***Glycerides** / *mono- and diglycerides* (GRAS)—Naturally occurring fats used as emulsifiers to maintain softness and consistency in dressings, gum, milk, ice cream, toppings, margarines, shortening, confections, and baked goods. Usually easily metabolized in the body and basically safe. The FDA is studying them for possible adverse effects.

***Glycerin** / *glycerol* (GRAS)—An alcohol found naturally in about 10 percent of animal and vegetable fats. In processed foods it is most often from animal sources. It is a solvent that helps carry food colors and flavors, a thickener in gelatin desserts, chewing gums and other processed foods, and a plasticizer used in the coverings for meats and cheeses. Also added to baked goods, bev-erages, and gelatinous meats. Glycerin is basically safe.

***Guar gum** (GRAS)—A complex carbohydrate, a sol-uble fiber extracted from the guar plant grown in the Middle East. It acts as a stabilizer, thickener, and binder in foods such as ice cream, cheese spreads, dressings, meat products, baked goods, and fruit drinks. There is some concern about its use by pregnant women, and large quantities may cause digestive upset in anyone. Otherwise it is safe.

***Gum Arabic**—*see Acacia*

***Honey** (GRAS)—Being used more commonly as a sweetener in many new natural, preservative-free bever-ages, cereals, ice creams, and candies. Honey contains both glucose and fructose and has less dramatic effects on blood sugar levels than cane sugar. It can be used directly from nature instead of being chemically extracted and processed. Honey is a safe food additive and actually has some preservative action. If used in excess, the calories and sugars can cause dental cavities and weight gain. Like all sugars, it is best used in moderation.

***HVP** / *hydrolyzed vegetable protein*—Used occasion-ally as a flavor enhancer in soups, gravies, and meats. It is also used in baby foods, although there is some con-cern about this, as HVP has the potential to affect the growth of children. Although HVP is still considered safe, I would avoid giving to young people.

***Iodine salts:** *calcium iodate, cuprous iodide, potas-sium iodate, and potassium iodide* (GRAS)—Iodine is a mineral that occurs naturally in the earth and sea and are needed by our body for proper thyroid function. Because iodine deficiency is common, potassium iodide is added to table salt to ensure that we receive our daily requirement.

Pregnant or lactating women usually require extra dietary iodine. Although iodine products can cause allergic reac-tions, the mineral is basically safe and is essential for life.

***Lactic acid** / *calcium lactate/butyl lactate/ethyl lac-tate* (GRAS)— Lactic acid is produced naturally in our body and in foods. Used to give flavor and tartness to beverages and to some desserts. Its acidity reduces spoilage in such foods as cheeses, olives, breads, butter, and candy. Helps condition dough and stabilize wine. Lactic acid is a safe additive.

***Lactose** / *milk sugar* (GRAS)—Occurs naturally in milk (about 5% concentration) and can be extracted from whey or during cheese making. Used in powdered infant formulas and protein powders for weight loss, weight gain, or body building; helps carry flavors and aromas in foods; and can improve the texture and flavor of baked goods. People who are lactose intolerant (lack the enzyme *lactase*, needed to break down lactose) may experience nausea, diarrhea, and bloating. For the majority of the population who tolerate dairy products, lactose is quite safe

**Lard and animal fats:* *pork fat, beef fat (tallow), cheese fat*—Fats from animals are commonly used in preparing soups and as flavoring additives. (These fats, especially lard, may be treated with unlisted chemicals and preserv-atives like BHT.) In small quantities, these animal fats are safe, but too much fat can cause cardiovascular disease. I suggest avoiding most animal fats and lard products.

***Lecithin** / *soy lecithin*—An oil found in most living tissues, lecithin is important to many body functions, particularly healthy nerves and cell membranes. Com-mercially, it is extracted from eggs, soybeans, or corn. Used mainly as an emulsifier and stabilizer in oil-con-taining foods, such as salad dressings, mayonnaise, mar-garine, chocolate, frozen desserts, cereals, and baked goods. Lecithin also acts as a mild antioxidant to pre-serve oil-containing products. Lecithin is safe and is reported to have beneficial effects.

***Locust bean gum**—*see Carob*

***Malic acid** (GRAS)—Occurs naturally in many fruits and vegetables, including apples, cherries, plums, and berries. Used to provide a tart taste to various sweets in wines, jams, sherbet, candies, beverages, and frozen milk products. It is basically safe, and studies show no poten-tial hazards.

***Malt/malt syrup** / *malt extract* (GRAS)—An extract from barley used commonly in the brewing industry and as a sweetener in foods, such as ice cream, flavored milk, candy, cereals, and dressings. Malt is safe, with no known toxicity.

***Maltol** / *synthetic ethyl maltol*—Not actually malt, but an extract from larch trees and pine needles, used as fla-voring to give foods a fresh-baked smell—in frozen desserts, gelatins, soft drinks, ice creams, candy, baked goods, and gums. Maltol is also known to be safe.

***Maple syrup**—a natural extract, this flavorful sweet-ener from maple trees is commonly used in place of sugar in many "health" foods. U.S. maple syrup manufacturers often use formaldehyde (a toxic chemical) on their trees to improve production; Canada does not allow formaldehyde. Many maple syrups are "imitations" and contain mostly sugar, corn syrup and artificial flavors with only a hint of actual maple syrup, and these are best avoided. Genuine maple syrup is a safe food, although excessive use should be avoided.

****Minerals**—Many are used to enrich and fortify foods. Examples are iron and calcium. Generally safe and often helpful. See Chapter 4 and chart on page 51 for more.

*MSG / Monosodium glutamate**—A controversial flavor enhancer that is extracted from molasses, used both in food processing (soups, spices, condiments, meats, and many Oriental foods), restaurant food, and as a seasoning for home cooking. It seems to speed up brain activity in unpredictable ways, with the potential for toxicity. Research has found that MSG caused brain tumors in baby mice, and has linked it with mood swings and depression. Animals fed MSG while pregnant had offspring that developed reproductive problems and reduced fertility as adults. "Chinese restaurant syndrome" from MSG has become associated with symptoms such as mild headaches in the temples, tingling, numbness, and chest pains. More research on MSG is needed. I suggest that we avoid foods containing MSG and restaurants that use it, particularly for children.

*Nitrites and Nitrates: sodium nitrite, potassium nitrite, sodium nitrate, potassium nitrate (saltpeter)**—Used in curing meats as a preservative (to prevent botulism) and color fixative in hams, bacon, sausage, hot dogs, corned beef, lunch meats, and some fish products. They add a tangy taste to the meats and prolong their shelf life. Nitrates and nitrites have been banned in Germany since 1977. They are considered unsafe, but still have not been banned in the U.S. Nitrate converts easily to nitrite, and the nitrites interact directly with natural ammonia byproducts in the digestive tract to form nitrosamines, which are highly carcinogenic chemicals. In animal studies, nitrosamines have been shown to cause cancer of the liver, lungs, and pancreas, all usually fatal conditions. Although nitrites are safer when used with vitamin C, my suggestion is to avoid all foods containing these substances, especially bacon, hot dogs, and cured meats, for obvious health reasons. If you do indulge in any of these questionable meats, take additional vitamin C and vitamin E when you do.

Oleic acid (GRAS)—Fatty acids obtained from animal and vegetable fats (safflower and olive oils). Used in food processing in making artificial butter, as a defoaming agent, and as a flavoring for beverages, desserts, and bakery products. Basically nontoxic in moderate amounts, but when it is hydrogenated, like any processed fat, it is best avoided.

*Olestra**—An oil polymer synthetic fake fat that is new and used initially in potato chips. It can cause common intestinal reactions. There has been much controversy in deciding to make it publicly available. At this time, I recommend avoiding Olestra.

Palmitic acid (GRAS)—Another fat found naturally in many animal and vegetable sources, such as butter, palm oil, and spices. Used to add a butter or cheese flavoring to seasoned foods. Basically nontoxic.

Parabens: methyl, butyl, and propyl paraben or parahydroxybenzoic acid—Synthetic compounds closely related to sodium benzoate, used as preservatives preventing the growth of molds and other microbes. Used in baked goods, desserts, and other processed foods. Fed in high amounts to experimental animals, they caused birth defects. If you wish to avoid synthetic chemicals with unknown effects, I would put the parabens in that class.

***Pectin** (GRAS)—A binding agent that occurs naturally in fruits and vegetables. A complex sugar extracted from the rinds and pressings of fruits, it is used in foods as a stabilizer and thickener to blend and gel jams, ice cream, desserts, beverages, and dressings. It is a safe food additive.

Polysorbate 60 and 80 / polyoxyethylene (20)/sorbitan monostearate/sorbitan monooleate (GRAS)—Derivatives made from sorbitol, a sugar-alcohol produced from glucose through the use of a toxic gas. Polysorbate 60 is an emulsifier that helps blend oil and water together and provides an even flavor in processed foods, such as salad dressings, dairy products, bakery goods, desserts, shortenings, whipped vegetable toppings, confections, and vitamin supplements. Polysorbate 80 is also used as an emulsifier and flavor carrier. There are some studies of possible toxicity, and I recommend avoidance or only occasional use.

Propyl gallate (GRAS)—A synthetic chemical added to foods for its antioxidant effect to prevent rancidity in foods containing fats and oils, such as in meats, shortenings, vegetable oils, snack foods, baked goods, and frozen dairy foods. Also used as flavoring in beverages, ice cream, candy, and bottled goods. Even though this chemical can be irritating in some people, propyl gallate is basically safe.

Propylene glycol / propylene glycol monostearate and alginate (GRAS)—A solvent blending agent made from propylene gas (a by-product of petroleum refining) and glycerol. Used in desserts and baked goods, in some salad dressings. These products have been shown to have very low toxicity, although they are still controversial chemicals and I would be wary of using their use.

Quinine / quinine hydrochloride / quinine sulfate (GRAS)—A bitter extract from the bark of the cinchona tree used to impart a refreshing bitter taste to carbonated beverages such as tonic water, bitter lemon, and quinine water. Quinine hydrochloride and sulfates are synthetic variations used as flavoring agents in beverages. Not recommended for use by pregnant women or people allergic to quinine. In general, small amounts are well tolerated.

Rennet / rennin—An enzyme extracted from the lining of the cow's stomach used to make cheese, as it helps to curdle milk. It has been found to be safe in the small amounts used. Many vegetarians prefer rennetless cheeses, which are made with vegetable enzymes.

*Saccharin / sodium saccharin—A popular artificial sweetener that contains no calories and is several hundred times sweeter than sugar, though it has a slightly bitter aftertaste. Saccharin has been found to cause bladder cancer in lab animals. In the second generation of animals fed saccharin, tumors occurred seven times more frequently than in animals not fed any saccharin. In 1977, the FDA tried to ban the use of saccharin in foods, but the public resisted the ban. Nearly five million pounds of saccharin have been used yearly—about 75 percent in diet drinks, 15 percent in other diet foods, and about 10 percent as a table sweetener. Since saccharin is not converted to glucose in the body, it is popular among diabetics. There is special risk to children, teenagers, and pregnant women. My current suggestion is not to use saccharin. It probably would be best to make saccharin available only by prescription.

** Salicylic acid and salicylates: amyl, phenyl, benzyl, and methyl salicylate—A number of foods, such as fruits, almonds, cucumbers, and tomatoes, contain natural salicylates. Salicylic acid, made synthetically by heating phenol with carbon dioxide, is the basis of aspirin (acetylsalicylic acid). Tartrazine, FDC Yellow #5, is a salicylate used as a food dye. The salicylates are also used in a variety of flavorings, such as strawberry and root beer in beverages, candies, baking goods, chewing gum, and ice cream. The higher doses of salicylates are known to cause ringing of the ears (tinnitus), gastrointestinal irritation, nausea, vomiting, increased respiration, acidosis, and skin rash. They are associated with food sensitivity in some children and adults with attention deficit disorder, who seem to function better on a diet free from salicylates.

** Silicates: silicon dioxide, sodium aluminosilicate, calcium and mangesium silicate, sodium calcium aluminosilicate, talc—Related to silicon, an important element relevant to bone development and connective tissue strength. Used as defoaming agents in beer production or as anticaking agents in salt, dry mixes, and baking powder. There are concerns about aluminum-containing silicates, and possible asbestos in talc; otherwise, the silicates are safe.

*Smoke flavoring / liquid smoke / char-smoke flavor—Manufactured by burning hardwoods such as maple or hickory. Used for flavoring, particularly meats and cheeses. Also mild antioxidants, protecting against fatty changes and helping to reduce bacteria. The benzopyrenes are suspected carcinogens, produced from the burning of the tars and resins in the wood. Until there is more research, I recommend avoiding these food additives.

**Sodium benzoate—see Benzoic acid

***Sodium bicarbonate / baking soda / bicarbonate of soda (GRAS)—An alkaline powder used to balance acid foods and to leaven and raise dough in many baking products, such as crackers, cake mixes, and muffins. Also

used as an antacid, as a substitute for toothpaste, and to absorb odors and freshen refrigerators. Sodium bicarbonate is a safe product.

*Sodium bisulfite—see Sulfites

**Sodium caseinate—see Caseinates

***Sodium chloride / "salt" / common table salt—A widely employed food additive in cooking and at the table, as a pickling and curing agent, as a mild preservative, and as a dough conditioner. Commercially extracted from salt mines or seawater, or through brine evaporation. Salt is basically safe when used in modest amounts. As a factor in causing high blood pressure, it is implicated in heart disease as well as in kidney disease. Unwise to consume in high amounts. (See *Staying Healthy With Nutrition,* Chapter 6.)

*Sodium nitrate and nitrite—see Nitrates; Nitrites

***Sorbic acid / potassium sorbate (GRAS)—A mild preservative used to inhibit bacteria and mold growth, especially in beverages, cheeses, and dessert products. Sorbic acid is basically safe and nontoxic, but it is still under review by the FDA.

**Sorbitan derivatives—see Polysorbate 60 and 80

**Sorbitol (GRAS)—A natural sugar found in fruits and sea vegetation that can be made chemically by modifying corn sugar (dextrose). Used to control crystallization as a thickener and texturizer in desserts, chewing gums, dietetic fruits and soft drinks. For diabetics, it is metabolized as a sugar. Thought to be safe, but it can be irritating to the intestinal tract. Ten grams (the amount in one candy bar) was found by researchers to cause diarrhea in children. Its use should be limited.

**Soy protein isolate / texturized vegetable protein (TVP)—A high-protein residue extracted from soybeans, used in milk-free formulas for infants, in protein-powder formulas for weight loss, weight gain, or body building as well as in soups, sauces, seasonings, meat substitutes, and processed foods. Can cause allergic responses such as intestinal upset, headache, or skin rashes. Since soy protein is not a complete food, it should not be consumed exclusively. Consult a doctor or nutritionist for weight-loss programs. In general, moderate amounts of the soy protein isolates are safe.

**Soy sauce / hydrolyzed and fermented soybeans—This is a salty food flavoring prepared by mold (usually Aspergillus) fermentation of soybeans. About 20 percent salt, it is used mainly in Oriental cooking. Soy sauce is safe but its salt content may be a disadvantage to those with high blood pressure or to people who are sensitive to mold-fermented products.

**Starches: acid-modified, modified, unmodified, gelatinized (GRAS)—A complex carbohydrate found in whole grains, vegetables, and tapioca, it can be used as a thickening or gelling agent in foods such as baby foods, gelatins, and cake mixes. Although safe, it is best to get our starches from whole foods and avoid most starch-added foods.

Stearic acid / calcium stearate (GRAS)—A saturated fatty acid from animal fats and hydrogenated vegetable oils. Used to lubricate or blend foods, in flavorings such as butter and vanilla, candies, chewing gum, and bakery products. Stearic acid may sensitize people to allergies. It caused tumors in experimental animals.

Succinic acid (GRAS)—Found naturally in meats and many vegetables with their distinct tart or acidic taste. Made synthetically by chemically changing acetic acid or maleic acid and used as a buffering or neutralizing agent, and to give an acid taste. Considered safe.

Sucrose (sugar made from sugar cane or beets)/white sugar/ refined sugar—The primary commercial and table sweetener in the U.S. It is a carbohydrate composed of glucose and fructose found in condiments (ketchup), dressings, candy, cereals, baby food, baked goods, desserts, and beverages, as well as vegetables, frozen meals, and most prepared meats. Sucrose is the number one food additive consumed by far. The average American consumes more than 125 pounds per year. Studies show that it is safe unless it is overconsumed or there is individual sensitivity. Overuse of sugar is implicated in adult-onset diabetes, obesity, hardening of the arteries and heart disease, low blood sugar, bacterial and yeast infections, mood swings and depression, and tooth decay. It is best to obtain our natural sugars from the many wholesome foods that contain them.

* **Sulfites:** *sodium sulfite, sodium and potassium bisulfite, sodium and potassium metabisulfite, sulfur dioxide* (GRAS)—Most of these sulfiting agents can release sulfur dioxide, which acts as a preservative and sanitizing agent. They prevent bacterial growth and the browning of exposed foods. Used in syrups and condiments, dried fruits and vegetables, and in wine making. Many people are allergic to sulfites. Those with a certain kind of asthma can actually go into anaphylactic shock, and at least seventeen deaths have been associated with its use. Sulfite reactions, including diarrhea, nausea, and headaches have also been reported. Sulfites are on my personal avoid list. Foods with the highest sulfite content are dried fruits and fruit juice concentrates, and wine, all of which you may want to buy organic.

Tannic acid (GRAS)—Found naturally in coffee and tea, wine, and the barks of certain trees. Used in beverages and desserts, as a clarifier in brewing, a refining agent for fats, and in flavorings (as an enjoyable astringent taste) like caramel, nut, maple, and others. Studies show it to be safe.

Tartaric acid (GRAS)—Found in grapes, wine, and other fruits, formed as a product of grape fermentation. Used to augment flavoring and to adjust acidity in beverages, baked goods, and desserts, and as a stabilizing agent to prevent color or flavor changes. Tartaric acid can be mildly irritating to the gastrointestinal tract in large doses. Studies show no toxicity.

TBHQ / tertiary butylhydroquinone—A butane gas derivative of petroleum, used to prevent rancidity of oils in combination with BHA or BHT. As little as 5 grams (a sixth of an ounce) has caused death. Ingestion of a single gram has caused nausea, vomiting, delirium, and collapse. I suggest avoiding this additive.

Vanilla (GRAS)—An aromatic and flavorful substance extracted from the vanilla bean, used as a flavoring in caramel, chocolate, root beer, butterscotch, butter, and some fruit flavorings for desserts and treats. It is very safe.

Vanillin (GRAS)—Vanillin and ethyl vanillin are stronger, synthetic analogues of vanilla, made from eugenol (an oil from cinnamon or cloves). This synthetic version of vanilla can be irritating. May be listed only as artificial or imitation flavoring. Use sparingly.

Vitamins—Many are used to enrich and fortify foods, when processing has removed them or the producer wants more nutients. Examples are riboflavin and folic acid. See Chapter 4 and the chart on page 51 for more information.

Whey / whey protein concentrate / milk serum (GRAS)—The liquid part of milk left after the casein is removed. Contains some milk protein and milk sugar (lactose). Can be dried to yield a mildly sweet powder that is used in cereals, ice cream, and dessert products, as an extender for meats, and in powdered nutritional supplements for weight control or body building. Basically safe, but people allergic to milk (the protein) or missing the lactase enzyme (lactose intolerant) often react to whey. Otherwise, well tolerated.

Xanthan gum (GRAS)—A complex carbohydrate made commercially by fermenting corn sugar with a bacteria. Used as an emulsifier and thickener in salad dressings, in dairy products, and in low-calorie foods. Tests show no hazards at even very high levels.

Xylitol—A simple alcohol carbohydrate made from wood sugar (xylose), a waste product of the wood-pulp industry. Not a true sugar, it is metabolized differently and is therefore usable for diabetics. It does not seem to promote dental decay (it may even help reduce cavities), so it is popular for use in chewing gums and found in other dietary foods and beverages. Safe in the amounts now used, but studies have suggested some long-term tumorigenic effects. Currently under review. Use only in moderation, not on a daily basis.

Yeasts: *baker's, brewer's, dried, torula yeast* (GRAS)—Single-cell fungi grown by the fermentation of carbohydrates. Yeast is high in nutrients, especially B vitamins, while dried yeast has some protein. Torula yeast is derived from Candida, grown on molasses or on petroleum by-products. Yeasts are found in soup mixes and gravies; condiments; and vitamin preparations. Smoked yeast should be avoided. Those sensitive to yeast may experience gas, bloating, or indigestion. People with an overgrowth of intestinal yeast should avoid all yeast-containing foods. Otherwise, a nutritious, safe, and useful additive.